MW00437774

A General Introduction to Psychoanalysis

BY
PROF. SIGMUND FREUD, LL.D.

AUTHORIZED TRANSLATION
WITH A PREFACE

BY
G. STANLEY HALL
PRESIDENT, CLARK UNIVERSITY

HORACE LIVERIGHT
PUBLISHER   NEW YORK

Published, 1920, by
HORACE LIVERIGHT, INC.

Printed in the United States of America
COPYRIGHT, 1920, BY EDWARD L. BERNAYS

PREFACE

Few, especially in this country, realize that while Freudian themes have rarely found a place on the programs of the American Psychological Association, they have attracted great and growing attention and found frequent elaboration by students of literature, history, biography, sociology, morals and aesthetics, anthropology, education, and religion. They have given the world a new conception of both infancy and adolescence, and shed much new light upon characterology; given us a new and clearer view of sleep, dreams, reveries, and revealed hitherto unknown mental mechanisms common to normal and pathological states and processes, showing that the law of causation extends to the most incoherent acts and even verbigerations in insanity; gone far to clear up the *terra incognita* of hysteria; taught us to recognize morbid symptoms, often neurotic and psychotic in their germ; revealed the operations of the primitive mind so overlaid and repressed that we had almost lost sight of them; fashioned and used the key of symbolism to unlock many mysticisms of the past; and in addition to all this, affected thousands of cures, established a new prophylaxis, and suggested new tests for character, disposition, and ability, in all combining the practical and theoretic to a degree salutary as it is rare.

These twenty-eight lectures to laymen are elementary and almost conversational. Freud sets forth with a frankness almost startling the difficulties and limitations of psychoanalysis, and also describes its main methods and results as only a master and originator of a new school of thought can do. These discourses are at the same time simple and almost confidential, and they trace and sum up the results of thirty years of devoted and painstaking research. While they are not at all controversial, we incidentally see in a clearer light the distinctions between the master and some of his distinguished pupils. A text like this is the most opportune and will naturally more or less supersede all other introductions to the general subject of psychoanalysis. It presents the author in a new light, as an effective and successful popularizer, and is certain to be welcomed not only by the large and growing number of students of psychoanalysis in this country but by the yet larger number of those who wish to begin its study here and elsewhere.

The impartial student of Sigmund Freud need not agree with all his conclusions, and indeed, like the present writer, may be unable to make sex so all-dominating a factor in the psychic life of the past and present as Freud deems it to be, to recognize the fact that he is the most original and creative mind in psychology of our generation. Despite the frightful handicap of the *odium sexicum*, far more formidable today than the *odium theologicum*, involving as it has done for him lack of academic recognition and even more or less social ostracism, his views have attracted and inspired a brilliant group of minds not only in psychiatry but in many other fields, who have altogether given the world of culture more new and pregnant *appercus* than those which have come from any other source within the wide domain of humanism.

A former student and disciple of Wundt, who recognizes to the full his inestimable services to our science, cannot avoid making certain comparisons. Wundt has had for decades the prestige of a most advantageous academic chair. He founded the first laboratory for experimental psychology, which attracted many of the most gifted and mature students from all lands. By his development of the doctrine of apperception he took psychology forever beyond the old associationism which had ceased to be fruitful. He also established the independence of psychology from physiology, and by his encyclopedic and always thronged lectures, to say nothing of his more or less esoteric seminary, he materially advanced every branch of mental science and extended its influence over the whole wide domain of folklore, mores, language, and primitive religion. His best texts will long constitute a thesaurus which every psychologist must know.

Again, like Freud, he inspired students who went beyond him (the Wurzburgers and introspectionists) whose method and results he could not follow. His limitations have grown more and more manifest. He has little use for the unconscious or the abnormal, and for the most part he has lived and wrought in a preevolutionary age and always and everywhere underestimated the genetic standpoint. He never transcends the conventional limits in dealing, as he so rarely does, with sex. Nor does he contribute much likely to be of permanent value in any part of the wide domain of affectivity. We cannot forbear to express the hope that Freud will not repeat Wundt's error in making too abrupt a break with his more advanced pupils like Adler or the Zurich group. It is rather precisely just the topics that Wundt neglects that Freud makes his chief corner-stones, viz., the unconscious, the abnormal, sex, and affectivity generally, with many genetic, especially ontogenetic, but also phylogenetic factors. The Wundtian influence has been great in the past, while Freud has a great present and a yet greater future.

In one thing Freud agrees with the introspectionists, viz., in deliberately neglecting the "physiological factor" and building on purely psychological foundations, although for Freud psychology is mainly unconscious, while for the introspectionists it is pure consciousness. Neither he nor his disciples have yet recognized the aid proffered them by students of the autonomic system or by the distinctions between the epicritic and protopathic functions and organs of the cerebrum, although these will doubtless come to have their due place as we know more of the nature and processes of the unconscious mind.

If psychologists of the normal have hitherto been too little disposed to recognize the precious contributions to psychology made by the cruel experiments of Nature in mental diseases, we think that the psychoanalysts, who work predominantly in this field, have been somewhat too ready to apply their findings to the operations of the normal mind; but we are optomistic enough to believe that in the end both these errors will vanish and that in the great synthesis of the future that now seems to impend our science will be made vastly richer and deeper on the theoretical side and also far more practical than it has ever been before.

G. Stanley Hall.

Clark   University,
   April, 1920.

CONTENTS

<u>PART ONE</u>

The Psychology of Errors

PAGE

PART TWO

The Dream

PART THREE

General Theory of the Neuroses

PART I

THE PSYCHOLOGY OF ERRORS

FIRST LECTURE

INTRODUCTION

I DO not know how familiar some of you may be, either from your reading or from hearsay, with psychoanalysis. But, in keeping with the title of these lectures—*A General Introduction to Psychoanalysis*—I am obliged to proceed as though you knew nothing about this subject, and stood in need of preliminary instruction.

To be sure, this much I may presume that you do know, namely, that psychoanalysis is a method of treating nervous patients medically. And just at this point I can give you an example to illustrate how the procedure in this field is precisely the reverse of that which is the rule in medicine. Usually when we introduce a patient to a medical technique which is strange to him we minimize its difficulties and give him confident promises concerning the result of the treatment. When, however, we undertake psychoanalytic treatment with a neurotic patient we proceed differently. We hold before him the difficulties of the method, its length, the exertions and the sacrifices which it will cost him; and, as to the result, we tell him that we make no definite promises, that the result depends on his conduct, on his understanding, on his adaptability, on his perseverance. We have, of course, excellent motives for conduct which seems so perverse, and into which you will perhaps gain insight at a later point in these lectures.

Do not be offended, therefore, if, for the present, I treat you as I treat these neurotic patients. Frankly, I shall dissuade you from coming to hear me a second time. With this intention I shall show what imperfections are necessarily involved in the teaching of psychoanalysis and what difficulties stand in the way of gaining a personal judgment. I shall show you how the whole trend of your previous training and all your accustomed mental habits must unavoidably have made you opponents of psychoanalysis, and how much you must overcome in yourselves in order to master this instinctive opposition. Of course I cannot predict how much psychoanalytic understanding you will gain from my lectures, but I can promise this, that by listening to them you will not learn how to undertake a psychoanalytic treatment or how to carry one to completion. Furthermore, should I find anyone among you who does not feel satisfied with a cursory acquaintance with psychoanalysis, but who would like to enter into a more enduring relationship with it, I shall not only dissuade him, but I shall actually warn him against it. As things now stand, a person would, by such a choice of profession, ruin his every chance of success at a university, and if he goes out into the world as a practicing physician, he will find himself in a society which does not understand his aims, which regards him with suspicion and hostility, and which turns loose upon him all the malicious spirits which lurk within it.

However, there are always enough individuals who are interested in anything which may be added to the sum total of knowledge, despite such inconveniences. Should there be any of this type among you, and should they ignore my dissuasion and return to the next of these lectures, they will be welcome. But all of you have the right to know what these difficulties of psychoanalysis are to which I have alluded.

First of all, we encounter the difficulties inherent in the teaching and exposition of psychoanalysis. In your medical instruction you have been accustomed to visual demonstration. You see the anatomical specimen, the precipitate in the chemical reaction, the contraction of the muscle as the result of the stimulation of its nerves. Later the patient is presented to your senses; the symptoms of his malady, the products of the pathological processes, in many cases even the cause of the disease is shown in isolated state. In the surgical department you are made to witness the steps by which one brings relief to the patient, and are permitted to attempt to practice them. Even in psychiatry, the demonstration affords you, by the patient's changed facial play, his manner of speech and his behavior, a wealth of observations which leave far-reaching impressions. Thus the medical teacher preponderantly plays the role of a guide and instructor who accompanies you through a museum in which you contract an immediate relationship to the exhibits, and in which you believe yourself to have been convinced through your own observation of the existence of the new things you see.

Unfortunately, everything is different in psychoanalysis. In psychoanalysis nothing occurs but the interchange of words between the patient and the physician. The patient talks, tells of his past experiences and present impressions, complains, confesses his wishes and emotions. The physician listens, tries to direct the thought processes of the patient, reminds him of things, forces his attention into certain channels, gives him explanations and observes the reactions of understanding or denial which he calls forth in the patient. The uneducated relatives of our patients—persons who are impressed only by the visible and tangible, preferably by such procedure as one sees in the moving picture theatres—never miss an opportunity of voicing their scepticism as to how one can "do anything for the malady through mere talk." Such thinking, of course, is as shortsighted as it is inconsistent. For these are the very persons who know with such certainty that the patients "merely imagine" their symptoms. Words were originally magic, and the word retains much of its old magical power even to-day. With words one man can make another blessed, or drive him to despair; by words the teacher transfers his knowledge to the pupil; by words the speaker sweeps his audience with him and determines its judgments and decisions. Words call forth effects and are the universal means of influencing human beings. Therefore let us not underestimate the use of words in psychotherapy, and let us be satisfied if we may be auditors of the words which are exchanged between the analyst and his patient.

But even that is impossible. The conversation of which the psychoanalytic treatment consists brooks no auditor, it cannot be demonstrated. One can, of course, present a neurasthenic or hysteric to the students in a psychiatric lecture.

He tells of his complaints and symptoms, but of nothing else. The communications which are necessary for the analysis are made only under the conditions of a special affective relationship to the physician; the patient would become dumb as soon as he became aware of a single impartial witness. For these communications concern the most intimate part of his psychic life, everything which as a socially independent person he must conceal from others; these communications deal with everything which, as a harmonious personality, he will not admit even to himself.

You cannot, therefore, "listen in" on a psychoanalytic treatment. You can only hear of it. You will get to know psychoanalysis, in the strictest sense of the word, only by hearsay. Such instruction even at second hand, will place you in quite an unusual position for forming a judgment. For it is obvious that everything depends on the faith you are able to put in the instructor.

Imagine that you are not attending a psychiatric, but an historical lecture, and that the lecturer is telling you about the life and martial deeds of Alexander the Great. What would be your reasons for believing in the authenticity of his statements? At first sight, the condition of affairs seems even more unfavorable than in the case of psychoanalysis, for the history professor was as little a participant in Alexander's campaigns as you were; the psychoanalyst at least tells you of things in connection with which he himself has played some role. But then the question turns on this—what set of facts can the historian marshal in support of his position? He can refer you to the accounts of ancient authors, who were either contemporaries themselves, or who were at least closer to the events in question; that is, he will refer you to the books of Diodor, Plutarch, Arrian, etc. He can place before you pictures of the preserved coins and statues of the king and can pass down your rows a photograph of the Pompeiian mosaics of the battle of Issos. Yet, strictly speaking, all these documents prove only that previous generations already believed in Alexander's existence and in the reality of his deeds, and your criticism might begin anew at this point. You will then find that not everything recounted of Alexander is credible, or capable of proof in detail; yet even then I cannot believe that you will leave the lecture hall a disbeliever in the reality of Alexander the Great. Your decision will be determined chiefly by two considerations; firstly, that the lecturer has no conceivable motive for presenting as truth something which he does not himself believe to be true, and secondly, that all available histories present the events in approximately the same manner. If you then proceed to the verification of the older sources, you will consider the same data, the possible motives of the writers and the consistency of the various parts of the evidence. The result of the examination will surely be convincing in the case of Alexander. It will probably turn out differently when applied to individuals like Moses and Nimrod. But what doubts you might raise against the credibility of the psychoanalytic reporter you will see plainly enough upon a later occasion.

At this point you have a right to raise the question, "If there is no such thing as objective verification of psychoanalysis, and no possibility of demonstrating it, how can one possibly learn psychoanalysis and convince himself of the truth of its claims?" The fact is, the study is not easy and there are not many persons who have learned psychoanalysis thoroughly; but nevertheless, there is a feasible way. Psychoanalysis is learned, first of all, from a study of one's self, through the study of one's own personality. This is not quite what is ordinarily called self-observation, but, at a pinch, one can sum it up thus. There is a whole series of very common and universally known psychic phenomena, which, after some instruction in the technique of psychoanalysis, one can make the subject matter of analysis in one's self. By so doing one obtains the desired conviction of the reality of the occurrences which psychoanalysis describes and of the correctness of its fundamental conception. To be sure, there are definite limits imposed on progress by this method. One gets much further if one allows himself to be analyzed by a competent analyst, observes the effect of the analysis on his own ego, and at the same time makes use of the opportunity to become familiar with the finer details of the technique of procedure. This excellent method is, of course, only practicable for one person, never for an entire class.

There is a second difficulty in your relation to psychoanalysis for which I cannot hold the science itself responsible, but for which I must ask you to take the responsibility upon yourselves, ladies and gentlemen, at least in so far as you have hitherto pursued medical studies. Your previous training has given your mental activity a definite bent which leads you far away from psychoanalysis. You have been trained to reduce the functions of an organism and its disorders anatomically, to explain them in terms of chemistry and physics and to conceive them biologically, but no portion of your interest has been directed to the psychic life, in which, after all, the activity of this wonderfully complex organism culminates. For this reason psychological thinking has remained strange to you and you have accustomed yourselves to regard it with suspicion, to deny it the character of the scientific, to leave it to the laymen, poets, natural philosophers and mystics. Such a delimitation is surely harmful to your medical activity, for the patient will, as is usual in all human relationships, confront you first of all with his psychic facade; and I am afraid your penalty will be this, that you will be forced to relinquish a portion of the therapeutic influence to which you aspire, to those lay physicians, nature-cure fakers and mystics whom you despise.

I am not overlooking the excuse, whose existence one must admit, for this deficiency in your previous training. There is no philosophical science of therapy which could be made practicable for your medical purpose. Neither speculative philosophy nor descriptive psychology nor that so-called experimental psychology which allies itself with the physiology of the sense organs as it is taught in the schools, is in a position to teach you anything useful concerning the relation between the physical and the psychical or to put into your hand the key to the understanding of a possible disorder of the psychic functions. Within the field of medicine, psychiatry does, it is true, occupy itself with the description of the observed psychic disorders and with their grouping into clinical symptom-pictures; but in their better hours the psychiatrists themselves doubt whether their purely descriptive account deserves the name of a science. The symptoms which constitute these clinical pictures are known neither in their origin, in their mechanism, nor in their mutual relationship. There are either no discoverable corresponding changes of the anatomical organ of the soul, or else the changes are of such a nature as to yield no enlightenment. Such psychic disturbances are open to therapeutic influence only when they can be identified as secondary phenomena of an otherwise organic affection.

Here is the gap which psychoanalysis aims to fill. It prepares to give psychiatry the omitted psychological foundation, it hopes to reveal the common basis from which, as a starting point, constant correlation of bodily and psychic disturbances becomes comprehensible. To this end, it must divorce itself from every anatomical, chemical or physiological supposition which is alien to it. It must work throughout with purely psychological therapeutic concepts, and just for that reason I fear that it will at first seem strange to you.

I will not make you, your previous training, or your mental bias share the guilt of the next difficulty. With two of its assertions, psychoanalysis offends the whole world and draws aversion upon itself. One of these assertions offends an intellectual prejudice, the other an aesthetic-moral one. Let us not think too lightly of these prejudices; they are powerful things, remnants of useful, even necessary, developments of mankind. They are retained through powerful affects, and the battle against them is a hard one.

The first of these displeasing assertions of psychoanalysis is this, that the psychic processes are in themselves unconscious, and that those which are conscious are merely isolated acts and parts of the total psychic life. Recollect that we are, on the contrary, accustomed to identify the psychic with the conscious. Consciousness actually means for us the distinguishing characteristic of the psychic life, and psychology is the science of the content of consciousness. Indeed, so obvious does this identification seem to us that we consider its slightest contradiction obvious nonsense, and yet psychoanalysis cannot avoid raising this contradiction; it cannot accept the identity of the conscious with the psychic. Its definition of the psychic affirms that they are processes of the nature of feeling, thinking, willing; and it must assert that there is such a thing as unconscious thinking and unconscious willing. But with this assertion psychoanalysis has alienated, to start with, the sympathy of all friends of sober science, and has laid itself open to the suspicion of being a fantastic mystery study which would build in darkness and fish in murky waters. You, however, ladies and gentlemen, naturally cannot as yet understand what justification I have for stigmatizing as a prejudice so abstract a phrase as this one, that "the psychic is consciousness." You cannot know what evaluation can have led to the denial of the unconscious, if such a thing really exists, and what advantage may have resulted from this denial. It sounds like a mere argument over words whether one shall say that the psychic coincides with the conscious or whether one shall extend it beyond that, and yet I can assure you that by the acceptance of unconscious processes you have paved the way for a decisively new orientation in the world and in science.

Just as little can you guess how intimate a connection this initial boldness of psychoanalysis has with the one which follows. The next assertion which psychoanalysis proclaims as one of its discoveries, affirms that those instinctive impulses which one can only call sexual in the narrower as well as in the wider sense, play an uncommonly large role in the causation of nervous and mental diseases, and that those impulses are a causation which has never been adequately appreciated. Nay, indeed, psychoanalysis claims that these same sexual impulses have made contributions whose value cannot be overestimated to the highest cultural, artistic and social achievements of the human mind.

According to my experience, the aversion to this conclusion of psychoanalysis is the most significant source of the opposition which it encounters. Would you like to know how we explain this fact? We believe that civilization was forged by the driving force of vital necessity, at the cost of instinct-satisfaction, and that the process is to a large extent constantly repeated anew, since each individual who newly enters the human community repeats the sacrifices of his instinct-satisfaction for the sake of the common good. Among the instinctive forces thus utilized, the sexual impulses play a significant role. They are thereby sublimated, i.e., they are diverted from their sexual goals and directed to ends socially higher and no longer sexual. But this result is unstable. The sexual instincts are poorly tamed. Each individual who wishes to ally himself with the achievements of civilization is exposed to the danger of having his sexual instincts rebel against this sublimation. Society can conceive of no more serious menace to its civilization than would arise through the satisfying of the sexual instincts by their redirection toward their original goals. Society, therefore, does not relish being reminded of this ticklish spot in its origin; it has no interest in having the strength of the sexual instincts recognized and the meaning of the sexual life to the individual clearly delineated. On the contrary, society has taken the course of diverting attention from this whole field. This is the reason why society will not tolerate the above-mentioned results of psychoanalytic research, and would prefer to brand it as aesthetically offensive and morally objectionable or dangerous. Since, however, one cannot attack an ostensibly objective result of scientific inquiry with such objections, the criticism must be translated to an intellectual level if it is to be voiced. But it is a predisposition of human nature to consider an unpleasant idea untrue, and then it is easy to find arguments against it. Society thus brands what is unpleasant as untrue, denying the conclusions of psychoanalysis with logical and pertinent arguments. These arguments originate from affective sources, however, and society holds to these prejudices against all attempts at refutation.

However, we may claim, ladies and gentlemen, that we have followed no bias of any sort in making any of these contested statements. We merely wished to state facts which we believe to have been discovered by toilsome labor. And we now claim the right unconditionally to reject the interference in scientific research of any such practical considerations, even before we have investigated whether the apprehension which these considerations are meant to instil are justified or not.

These, therefore, are but a few of the difficulties which stand in the way of your occupation with psychoanalysis. They are perhaps more than enough for a beginning. If you can overcome their deterrent impression, we shall continue.

SECOND LECTURE

THE PSYCHOLOGY OF ERRORS

W E begin with an investigation, not with hypotheses. To this end we choose certain phenomena which are very frequent, very familiar and very little heeded, and which have nothing to do with the pathological, inasmuch as they can be observed in every normal person. I refer to the errors which an individual commits—as for example, errors of speech in which he wishes to say something and uses the wrong word; or those which happen to him in writing, and which he may or may not notice; or the case of misreading, in which one reads in the print or writing something different from what is actually there. A similar phenomenon occurs in those cases of mishearing what is said to one, where there is no question of an organic disturbance of the auditory function. Another series of such occurrences is based on forgetfulness—but on a forgetfulness which is not permanent, but temporary, as for instance when one cannot think of a name which one knows and always recognizes; or when one forgets to carry out a project at the proper time but which one remembers again later, and therefore has only forgotten for a certain interval. In a third class this characteristic of transience is lacking, as for example in mislaying things so that they cannot be found again, or in the analogous case of losing things. Here we are dealing with a kind of forgetfulness to which one reacts differently from the other cases, a forgetfulness at which one is surprised and annoyed, instead of considering it comprehensible. Allied with these phenomena is that of erroneous ideas—in which the element of transience is again prominent, inasmuch as for a while one believes something which, before and after that time, one knows to be untrue—and a number of similar phenomena of different designations.

These are all occurrences whose inner connection is expressed in the use of the same prefix of designation.[1] They are almost all unimportant, generally temporary and without much significance in the life of the individual. It is only rarely that one of them, such as the phenomenon of losing things, attains to a certain practical importance. For that reason also they do not attract much attention, they arouse only weak affects.

It is, therefore, to these phenomena that I would now direct your attention. But you will object, with annoyance: "There are so many sublime riddles in the external world, just as there are in the narrower world of the psychic life, and so many wonders in the field of psychic disturbances which demand and deserve elucidation, that it really seems frivolous to waste labor and interest on such trifles. If you can explain to us how an individual with sound eyes and ears can, in broad daylight, see and hear things that do not exist, or why another individual suddenly believes himself persecuted by those whom up to that time he loved best, or defend, with the most ingenious arguments, delusions which must seem nonsense to any child, then we will be willing to consider psychoanalysis seriously. But if psychoanalysis can do nothing better than to occupy us with the question of why a speaker used the wrong word, or why a housekeeper mislaid her keys, or such trifles, then we know something better to do with our time and interest."

My reply is: "Patience, ladies and gentlemen. I think your criticism is not on the right track. It is true that psychoanalysis cannot boast that it has never occupied itself with trifles. On the contrary, the objects of its observations are generally those simple occurrences which the other sciences have thrown aside as much too insignificant, the waste products of the phenomenal world. But are you not confounding, in your criticism, the sublimity of the problems with the conspicuousness of their manifestations? Are there not very important things which under certain circumstances, and at certain times, can betray themselves only by very faint signs? I could easily cite a great many instances of this kind. From what vague signs, for instance, do the young gentlemen of this audience conclude that they have won the favor of a lady? Do you await an explicit declaration, an ardent embrace, or does not a glance, scarcely perceptible to others, a fleeting gesture, the prolonging of a hand-shake by one second, suffice? And if you are a criminal lawyer, and engaged in the investigation of a murder, do you actually expect the murderer to leave his photograph and address on the scene of the crime, or would you, of necessity, content yourself with fainter and less certain traces of that individual? Therefore, let us not undervalue small signs; perhaps by means of them we will succeed in getting on the track of greater things. I agree with you that the larger problems of the world and of science have the first claim on our interest. But it is generally of little avail to form the definite resolution to devote oneself to the investigation of this or that problem. Often one does not know in which direction to take the next step. In scientific research it is more fruitful to attempt what happens to be before one at the moment and for whose investigation there is a discoverable method. If one does that thoroughly without prejudice or predisposition, one may, with good fortune, and by virtue of the connection which links each thing to every other (hence also the small to the great) discover even from such modest research a point of approach to the study of the big problems."

Thus would I answer, in order to secure your attention for the consideration of these apparently insignificant errors made by normal people. At this point, we will question a stranger to psychoanalysis and ask him how he explains these occurrences.

His first answer is sure to be, "Oh, they are not worth an explanation; they are merely slight accidents." What does he mean by this? Does he mean to assert that there are any occurrences so insignificant that they fall out of the causal sequence of things, or that they might just as well be something different from what they are? If any one thus denies the determination of natural phenomena at one such point, he has vitiated the entire scientific viewpoint. One can then point out to him how much more consistent is the religious point of view, when it explicitly asserts that "No sparrow falls from the roof without God's special wish." I imagine our friend will not be willing to follow his first answer to its logical conclusion; he will interrupt and say that if he were to study these things he would probably find an explanation for them. He will say that this is a case of slight functional disturbance, of an inaccurate psychic act whose causal factors can be outlined. A man who otherwise speaks correctly may make a slip of the tongue—when he is slightly ill or fatigued; when he is excited; when his attention is concentrated on something else. It is easy to prove these statements. Slips of the tongue do really occur with special frequency when one is tired, when one has a headache or when one is indisposed. Forgetting proper names is a very frequent occurrence under these circumstances. Many persons even recognize the imminence of an indisposition by the inability to recall proper names. Often also one mixes up words or objects during excitement, one picks up the wrong things; and the forgetting of projects, as well as the doing of any number of other unintentional acts, becomes conspicuous when one is distracted; in other words, when one's attention is concentrated on other things. A familiar instance of such distraction is the professor in *Fliegende Blätter*, who takes the wrong hat because he is thinking of the problems which he wishes to treat in his next book. Each of us knows from experience some examples of how one can forget projects which one has planned and promises which one has made, because an experience has intervened which has preoccupied one deeply.

This seems both comprehensible and irrefutable. It is perhaps not very interesting, not as we expected it to be. But let us consider this explanation of errors. The conditions which have been cited as necessary for the occurrence of these phenomena are not all identical. Illness and disorders of circulation afford a physiological basis. Excitement, fatigue and distraction are conditions of a different sort, which one could designate as psycho-physiological. About these latter it is easy to theorize. Fatigue, as well as distraction, and perhaps also general excitement, cause a scattering of the attention which can result in the act in progress not receiving sufficient attention. This act can then be more easily interrupted than usual, and may be inexactly carried out. A slight illness, or a change in the distribution of blood in the central organ of the nervous system, can have the same effect, inasmuch as it influences the determining factor, the distribution of attention, in a similar way. In all cases, therefore, it is a question of the effects of a distraction of the attention, caused either by organic or psychic factors.

But this does not seem to yield much of interest for our psychoanalytic investigation. We might even feel tempted to give up the subject. To be sure, when we look more closely wefind that not everything squares with this attention theory of psychological errors, or that at any rate not everything can be directly deduced from it. We find that such errors and such forgetting occur even when people are not fatigued, distracted or excited, but are in every way in their normal state; unless, in consequence of these errors, one were to attribute to them an excitement which they themselves do not acknowledge. Nor is the mechanism so simple that the success of an act is assured by an intensification of the attention bestowed upon it, and endangered by its diminution. There are many acts which one performs in a purely automatic way and with very little attention, but which are yet carried out quite successfully. The pedestrian who scarcely knows where he is going, nevertheless keeps to the right road and stops at his destination without having gone astray. At least, this is the rule. The practiced pianist touches the right keys without thinking of them. He may, of course, also make an occasional mistake, but if automatic playing increased the likelihood of errors, it would be just the virtuoso whose playing has, through practice, become most automatic, who would be the most exposed to this danger. Yet we see, on the contrary, that many acts are most successfully carried out when they are not the objects of particularly concentrated attention, and that the mistakes occur just at the point where one is most anxious to be accurate—where a distraction of the necessary attention is therefore surely least permissible. One could then say that this is the effect of the "excitement," but we do not understand why the excitement does not intensify the concentration of attention on the goal that is so much desired. If in an important speech or discussion anyone says the opposite of what he means, then that can hardly be explained according to the psycho-physiological or the attention theories.

There are also many other small phenomena accompanying these errors, which are not understood and which have not been rendered comprehensible to us by these explanations. For instance, when one has temporarily forgotten a name, one is annoyed, one is determined to recall it and is unable to give up the attempt. Why is it that despite his annoyance the individual cannot succeed, as he wishes, in directing his attention to the word which is "on the tip of his tongue," and which he instantly recognizes when it is pronounced to him? Or, to take another example, there are cases in which the errors multiply, link themselves together, substitute for each other. The first time one forgets an appointment; the next time, after having made a special resolution not to forget it, one discovers that one has made a mistake in the day or hour. Or one tries by devious means to remember a forgotten word, and in the course of so doing loses track of a second name which would have been of use in finding the first. If one then pursues this second name, a third gets lost, and so on. It is notorious that the same thing can happen in the case of misprints, which are of course to be considered as errors of the typesetter. A stubborn error of this sort is said to have crept into a Social-Democratic paper, where, in the account of a certain festivity was printed, "Among those present was His Highness, the Clown Prince." The next day a correction was attempted. The paper apologized and said, "The sentence should, of course, have read 'The Clown Prince.'" One likes to attribute these occurrences to the printer's devil, to the goblin of the typesetting machine, and the like—figurative expressions which at least go beyond a psycho-physiological theory of the misprint.

I do not know if you are acquainted with the fact that one can provoke slips of the tongue, can call them forth by suggestion, as it were. An anecdote will serve to illustrate this. Once when a novice on the stage was entrusted with the important role in *The Maid of Orleans* of announcing to the King, "Connétable sheathes his sword," the star played the joke of repeating to the frightened beginner during the rehearsal, instead of the text, the following, "Comfortable sends back his steed,"[2] and he attained his end. In the performance the unfortunate actor actually made his début with this distorted announcement; even after he had been amply warned against so doing, or perhaps just for that reason.

These little characteristics of errors are not exactly illuminated by the theory of diverted attention. But that does not necessarily prove the whole theory wrong. There is perhaps something missing, a complement by the addition of which the theory would be made completely satisfactory. But many of the errors themselves can be regarded from another aspect.

Let us select slips of the tongue, as best suited to our purposes. We might equally well choose slips of the pen or of reading. But at this point, we must make clear to ourselves the fact that so far we have inquired only as to when and under what conditions one's tongue slips, and have received an answer on this point only. One can, however, direct one's interest elsewhere and ask why one makes just this particular slip and no other; one can consider what the slip results in. You must realize that as long as one does not answer this question—does not explain the effect produced by the slip—the phenomenon in its psychological aspect remains an accident, even if its physiological explanation has been found. When it happens that I commit a slip of the tongue, I could obviously make any one of an infinite number of slips, and in place of the one right word say any one of a thousand others, make innumerable distortions of the right word. Now, is there anything which forces upon me in a specific instance just this one special slip out of all those which are possible, or does that remain accidental and arbitrary, and can nothing rational be found in answer to this question?

Two authors, Meringer and Mayer (a philologist and a psychiatrist) did indeed in 1895 make the attempt to approach the problem of slips of the tongue from this side. They collected examples and first treated them from a purely descriptive standpoint. That, of course, does not yet furnish any explanation, but may open the way to one. They differentiated the distortions which the intended phrase suffered through the slip, into: interchanges of positions of words, interchanges of parts of words, perseverations, compoundings and substitutions. I will give you examples of these authors' main categories. It is a case of interchange of the first sort if someone says "the Milo of Venus" instead of "the Venus of Milo." An example of the second type of interchange, "I had a blush of rood to the head" instead of "rush of blood"; a perseveration would be the familiar misplaced toast, "I ask you to join me in hiccoughing the health of our chief."[3] These three forms of slips are not very frequent. You will find those cases much more frequent in which the slip results from a drawing together or compounding of syllables; for example, a gentleman on the street addresses a lady with the words, "If you will allow me, madame, I should be very glad to *inscort* you."[4] In the compounded word there is obviously besides the word "escort," also the word "insult" (and parenthetically we may remark that the young man will not find much favor with the lady). As an example of the substitution, Meringer and Mayer cite the following: "A man says, 'I put the specimens in the letterbox,' instead of 'in the hot-bed,' and the like."[5]

The explanation which the two authors attempt to formulate on the basis of this collection of examples is peculiarly inadequate. They hold that the sounds and syllables of words have different values, and that the production and perception of more highly valued syllables can interfere with those of lower values. They obviously base this conclusion on the cases of fore-sounding and perseveration which are not at all frequent; in other cases of slips of the tongue the question of such sound priorities, if any exist, does not enter at all. The most frequent cases of slips of the tongue are those in which instead of a certain word one says another which resembles it; and one may consider this resemblance sufficient explanation. For example, a professor says in his initial lecture, "I am not *inclined* to evaluate the merits of my predecessor."[6] Or another professor says, "In the case of the female genital, despite many *temptations* ... I mean many attempts ... etc."[7]

The most common, and also the most conspicuous form of slips of the tongue, however, is that of saying the exact opposite of what one meant to say. In such cases, one goes far afield from the problem of sound relations and resemblance effects, and can cite, instead of these, the fact that opposites have an obviously close relationship to each other, and have particularly close relations in the psychology of association. There are historical examples of this sort. A president of our House of Representatives once opened the assembly with the words, "Gentlemen, I declare a quorum present, and herewith declare the assembly *closed.*"

Similar, in its trickiness, to the relation of opposites is the effect of any other facile association which may under certain circumstances arise most inopportunely. Thus, for instance, there is the story which relates that on the occasion of a festivity in honor of the marriage of a child of H. Helmholtz with a child of the well-known discoverer and captain of industry, W. Siemon, the famous physiologist Dubois-Reymond was asked to speak. He concluded his undoubtedly sparkling toast with the words, "Success to the new firm—Siemens and—Halski!" That, of course, was the name of the well-known old firm. The association of the two names must have been about as easy for a native of Berlin as "Weber and Fields" to an American.

Thus we must add to the sound relations and word resemblances the influence of word associations. But that is not all. In a series of cases, an explanation of the observed slip is unsuccessful unless we take into account what phrase had been said or even thought previously. This again makes it a case of perseveration of the sort stressed by Meringer, but of a longer duration. I must admit, I am on the whole of the impression that we are further than ever from an explanation of slips of the tongue!

However, I hope I am not wrong when I say that during the above investigation of these examples of slips of the tongue, we have all obtained a new impression on which it will be of value to dwell. We sought the general conditions under which slips of the tongue occur, and then the influences which determine the kind of distortion resulting from the slip, but we have in no way yet considered the effect of the slip of the tongue in itself, without regard to its origin. And if we should decide to do so we must finally have the courage to assert, "In some of the examples cited, the product of the slip also makes sense." What do we mean by "it makes sense"? It means, I think, that the product of the slip has itself a right to be considered as a valid psychic act which also has its purpose, as a manifestation having content and meaning. Hitherto we have always spoken of errors, but now it seems as if sometimes the error itself were quite a normal act, except that it has thrust itself into the place of some other expected or intended act.

In isolated cases this valid meaning seems obvious and unmistakable. When the president with his opening words closes the session of the House of Representatives, instead of opening it, we are inclined to consider this error meaningful by reason of our knowledge of the circumstances under which the slip occurred. He expects no good of the assembly, and would be glad if he could terminate it immediately. The pointing out of this meaning, the interpretation of this error, gives us no difficulty. Or a lady, pretending to admire, says to another, "I am sure you must have messed up this charming hat yourself."[8] No scientific quibbles in the world can keep us from discovering in this slip the idea "this hat is a mess." Or a lady who is known for her energetic disposition, relates, "My husband asked the doctor to what diet he should keep. But the doctor said he didn't need any diet, he should eat and drink whatever *I* want." This slip of tongue is quite an unmistakable expression of a consistent purpose.

Ladies and gentlemen, if it should turn out that not only a few cases of slips of the tongue and of errors in general, but the larger part of them, have a meaning, then this meaning of errors of which we have hitherto made no mention, will unavoidably become of the greatest interest to us and will, with justice, force all other points of view into the background. We could then ignore all physiological and psycho-physiological conditions and devote ourselves to the purely psychological investigations of the sense, that is, the meaning, the purpose of these errors. To this end therefore we will not fail, shortly, to study a more extensive compilation of material.

But before we undertake this task, I should like to invite you to follow another line of thought with me. It has repeatedly happened that a poet has made use of slips of the tongue or some other error as a means of poetic presentation. This fact in itself must prove to us that he considers the error, the slip of the tongue for instance, as meaningful; for he creates it on purpose, and it is not a case of the poet committing an accidental slip of the pen and then letting his pen-slip stand as a tongue-slip of his character. He wants to make something clear to us by this slip of the tongue, and we may examine what it is, whether he wishes to indicate by this that the person in question is distracted or fatigued. Of course, we do not wish to exaggerate the importance of the fact that the poet did make use of a slip to express his meaning. It could nevertheless really be a psychic accident, or meaningful only in very rare cases, and the poet would still retain the right to infuse it with meaning through his setting. As to their poetic use, however, it would not be surprising if we should glean more information concerning slips of the tongue from the poet than from the philologist or the psychiatrist.

Such an example of a slip of the tongue occurs in *Wallenstein* (*Piccolomini*, Act 1, Scene 5). In the previous scene, Max Piccolomini has most passionately sided with the Herzog, and dilated ardently on the blessings of peace which disclosed themselves to him during the trip on which he accompanied Wallenstein's daughter to the camp. He leaves his father and the courtier, Questenberg, plunged in deepest consternation. And then the fifth scene continues:

Q.

    Alas! Alas! and stands it so?

    What friend! and do we let him go away

    In this delusion—let him go away?

    Not call him back immediately, not open

    His eyes upon the spot?

Octavio.

        (*Recovering himself out of a deep study*)

    He has now opened mine,

    And I see more than pleases me.

Q.

What is it?

OCTAVIO.

A curse on this journey!

Q.

But why so? What is it?

OCTAVIO.

Come, come along, friend! I must follow up

The ominous track immediately. Mine eyes

Are opened now, and I must use them. Come!

(*Draws Q. on with him.*)

Q.

What now? Where go you then?

OCTAVIO.

(*Hastily.*) To *her* herself

Q.

To—

OCTAVIO.

(*Interrupting him and correcting himself.*)

To the duke. Come, let us go—.

Octavio meant to say, "To him, to the lord," but his tongue slips and through his words "*to her*" he betrays to us, at least, the fact that he had quite clearly recognized the influence which makes the young war hero dream of peace.

A still more impressive example was found by O. Rank in Shakespeare. It occurs in the *Merchant of Venice*, in the famous scene in which the fortunate suitor makes his choice among the three caskets; and perhaps I can do no better than to read to you here Rank's short account of the incident:

"A slip of the tongue which occurs in Shakespeare's *Merchant of Venice*, Act III, Scene II, is exceedingly delicate in its poetic motivation and technically brilliant in its handling. Like the slip in *Wallenstein* quoted by Freud (*Psychopathology of Everyday Life*, 2d ed., p. 48), it shows that the poets well know the meaning of these errors and assume their comprehensibility to the audience. Portia, who by her father's wish has been bound to the choice of a husband by lot, has so far escaped all her unfavored suitors through the fortunes of chance. Since she has finally found in Bassanio the suitor to whom she is attached, she fears that he, too, will choose the wrong casket. She would like to tell him that even in that event he may rest assured of her love, but is prevented from so doing by her oath. In this inner conflict the poet makes her say to the welcome suitor:

PORTIA:

I pray you tarry; pause a day or two,

Before you hazard; for, in choosing wrong

I lose your company; therefore, forbear a while:

There's something tells me, (but it is not love)

I would not lose you: * * *

* * * I could teach you

How to choose right, but then I am forsworn,

So will I never be: so may you miss me;

But if you do, you'll make me wish a sin

That I had been forsworn. Beshrew your eyes.

They have o'erlook'd me, and divided me;

One half of me is yours, the other half *yours*,

Mine own, I would say: but if mine, then yours,

And so all yours.

Just that, therefore, which she meant merely to indicate faintly to him or really to conceal from him entirely, namely that even before the choice of the lot she was his and loved him, this the poet—with admirable psychological delicacy of feeling—makes apparent by her slip; and is able, by this artistic device, to quiet the unbearable uncertainty of the lover, as well as the equal suspense of the audience as to the issue of the choice."

Notice, at the end, how subtly Portia reconciles the two declarations which are contained in the slip, how she resolves the contradiction between them and finally still manages to keep her promise:

"* * * but if mine, then yours,

And so all yours."

Another thinker, alien to the field of medicine, accidentally disclosed the meaning of errors by an observation which has anticipated our attempts at explanation. You all know the clever satires of Lichtenberg (1742-1749), of which Goethe said, "Where he jokes, there lurks a problem concealed." Not infrequently the joke also brings to light the solution of the problem. Lichtenberg mentions in his jokes and satiric comments the remark that he always read "Agamemnon" for "angenommen,"[9] so intently had he read Homer. Herein is really contained the whole theory of misreadings.

At the next session we will see whether we can agree with the poets in their conception of the meaning of psychological errors.

THIRD LECTURE

THE PSYCHOLOGY OF ERRORS—(*Continued*)

AT the last session we conceived the idea of considering the error, not in its relation to the intended act which it distorted, but by itself alone, and we received the impression that in isolated instances it seems to betray a meaning of its own. We declared that if this fact could be established on a larger scale, then the meaning of the error itself would soon come to interest us more than an investigation of the circumstances under which the error occurs.

Let us agree once more on what we understand by the "meaning" of a psychic process. A psychic process is nothing more than the purpose which it serves and the position which it holds in a psychic sequence. We can also substitute the word "purpose" or "intention" for "meaning" in most of our investigations. Was it then only a deceptive appearance or a poetic exaggeration of the importance of an error which made us believe that we recognized a purpose in it?

Let us adhere faithfully to the illustrative example of slips of the tongue and let us examine a larger number of such observations. We then find whole categories of cases in which the intention, the meaning of the slip itself, is clearly manifest. This is the case above all in those examples in which one says the opposite of what one intended. The president said, in his opening address, "I declare the meeting closed." His intention is certainly not ambiguous. The meaning and purpose of his slip is that he wants to terminate the meeting. One might point the conclusion with the remark "he said so himself." We have only taken him at his word. Do not interrupt me at this point by remarking that this is not possible, that we know he did not want to terminate the meeting but to open it, and that he himself, whom we have just recognized as the best judge of his intention, will affirm that he meant to open it. In so doing you forget that we have agreed to consider the error entirely by itself. Its relation to the intention which it distorts is to be discussed later. Otherwise you convict yourself of an error in logic by which you smoothly conjure away the problem under discussion; or "beg the question," as it is called in English.

In other cases in which the speaker has not said the exact opposite of what he intended, the slip may nevertheless express an antithetical meaning. "I am not *inclined* to appreciate the merits of my predecessor." "*Inclined*" is not the opposite of "*in a position to*," but it is an open betrayal of intent in sharpest contradiction to the attempt to cope gracefully with the situation which the speaker is supposed to meet.

In still other cases the slip simply adds a second meaning to the one intended. The sentence then sounds like a contradiction, an abbreviation, a condensation of several sentences. Thus the lady of energetic disposition, "He may eat and drink whatever *I* please." The real meaning of this abbreviation is as though the lady had said, "He may eat and drink whatever he pleases. But what does it matter what *he* pleases! It is *I* who do the pleasing." Slips of the tongue often give the impression of such an abbreviation. For example, the anatomy professor, after his lecture on the human nostril, asks whether the class has thoroughly understood, and after a unanimous answer in the affirmative, goes on to say: "I can hardly believe that is so, since the people who understand the human nostril can, even in a city of millions, be counted on *one finger*—I mean, on the fingers of one hand." The abbreviated sentence here also has its meaning: it expresses the idea that there is only one person who thoroughly understands the subject.

In contrast to these groups of cases are those in which the error does not itself express its meaning, in which the slip of the tongue does not in itself convey anything intelligible; cases, therefore, which are in sharpest opposition to our expectations. If anyone, through a slip of the tongue, distorts a proper name, or puts together an unusual combination of syllables, then this very common occurrence seems already to have decided in the negative the question of whether all errors contain a meaning. Yet closer inspection of these examples discloses the fact that an understanding of such a distortion is easily possible, indeed, that the difference between these unintelligible cases and the previous comprehensible ones is not so very great.

A man who was asked how his horse was, answered, "Oh, it may *stake*—it may take another month." When asked what he really meant to say, he explained that he had been thinking that it was a *sorry* business and the coming together of "*take*" and "*sorry*" gave rise to "*stake*." (Meringer and Mayer.)

Another man was telling of some incidents to which he had objected, and went on, "and then certain facts were *re-filed*." Upon being questioned, he explained that he meant to stigmatize these facts as "*filthy*." "*Revealed*" and "*filthy*" together produced the peculiar "*re-filled*." (Meringer and Mayer.)

You will recall the case of the young man who wished to "*inscort*" an unknown lady. We took the liberty of resolving this word construction into the two words "*escort*" and "*insult*," and felt convinced of this interpretation without demanding proof of it. You see from these examples that even slips can be explained through the concurrence, the interference, of two speeches of different intentions. The difference arises only from the fact that in the one type of slip the intended speech completely crowds out the other, as happens in those slips where the opposite is said, while in the other type the intended speech must rest content with so distorting or modifying the other as to result in mixtures which seem more or less intelligible in themselves.

We believe that we have now grasped the secret of a large number of slips of the tongue. If we keep this explanation in mind we will be able to understand still other hitherto mysterious groups. In the case of the distortion of names, for instance, we cannot assume that it is always an instance of competition between two similar, yet different names. Still, the second intention is not difficult to guess. The distorting of names occurs frequently enough not as a slip of the tongue, but as an attempt to give the name an ill-sounding or debasing character. It is a familiar device or trick of insult, which persons of culture early learned to do without, though they do not give it up readily. They often clothe it in the form of a joke, though, to be sure, the joke is of a very low order. Just to cite a gross and ugly example of such a distortion of a name, I mention the fact that the name of the President of the French Republic, *Poincaré*, has been at times, lately, transformed into "*Schweinskarré*." It is therefore easy to assume that there is also such an intention to insult in the case of other slips of the tongue which result in the distortion of a name. In consequence of our adherence to this conception, similar explanations force themselves upon us, in the case of slips of the tongue whose effect is comical or absurd. "I call upon you to *hiccough* the health of our chief."[10] Here the solemn atmosphere is unexpectedly disturbed by the introduction of a word that awakens an unpleasant image; and from the prototype of certain expressions of insult and offense we cannot but suppose that there is an intention striving for expression which is in sharp contrast to the ostensible respect, and which could be expressed about as follows, "You needn't believe this. I'm not really in earnest. I don't give a whoop for the fellow—etc." A similar trick which passes for a slip of the tongue is that which transforms a harmless word into one which is indecent and obscene.[11]

We know that many persons have this tendency of intentionally making harmless words obscene for the sake of a certain lascivious pleasure it gives them. It passes as wit, and we always have to ask about a person of whom we hear such a thing, whether he intended it as a joke or whether it occurred as a slip of the tongue.

Well, here we have solved the riddle of errors with relatively little trouble! They are not accidents, but valid psychic acts. They have their meaning; they arise through the collaboration—or better, the mutual interference—of two different intentions. I can well understand that at this point you want to swamp me with a deluge of questions and doubts to be answered and resolved before we can rejoice over this first result of our labors. I truly do not wish to push you to premature conclusions. Let us dispassionately weigh each thing in turn, one after the other.

What would you like to say? Whether I think this explanation is valid for all cases of slips of the tongue or only for a certain number? Whether one can extend this same conception to all the many other errors—to mis-reading, slips of the pen, forgetting, picking up the wrong object, mislaying things, etc? In the face of the psychic nature of errors, what meaning is left to the factors of fatigue, excitement, absent-mindedness and distraction of attention? Moreover, it is easy to see that of the two competing meanings in an error, one is always public, but the other not always. But what does one do in order to guess the latter? And when one believes one has guessed it, how does one go about proving that it is not merely a probable meaning, but that it is the only correct meaning? Is there anything else you wish to ask? If not, then I will continue. I would remind you of the fact that we really are not much concerned with the errors themselves, but we wanted only to learn something of value to psychoanalysis from their study. Therefore, I put the question: What are these purposes or tendencies which can thus interfere with others, and what relation is there between the interfering tendencies and those interfered with? Thus our labor really begins anew, after the explanation of the problem.

Now, is this the explanation of all tongue slips? I am very much inclined to think so and for this reason, that as often as one investigates a case of a slip of the tongue, it reduces itself to this type of explanation. But on the other hand, one cannot prove that a slip of the tongue cannot occur without this mechanism. It may be so; for our purposes it is a matter of theoretical indifference, since the conclusions which we wish to draw by way of an introduction to psychoanalysis remain untouched, even if only a minority of the cases of tongue slips come within our conception, which is surely not the case. I shall anticipate the next question, of whether or not we may extend to other types of errors what we have gleaned from slips of the tongue, and answer it in the affirmative. You will convince yourselves of that conclusion when we turn our attention to the investigation of examples of pen slips, picking up wrong objects, etc. I would advise you, however, for technical reasons, to postpone this task until we shall have investigated the tongue slip itself more thoroughly.

The question of what meaning those factors which have been placed in the foreground by some authors,—namely, the factors of circulatory disturbances, fatigue, excitement, absent-mindedness, the theory of the distraction of attention— the question of what meaning those factors can now have for us if we accept the above described psychic mechanism of tongue slips, deserves a more detailed answer. You will note that we do not deny these factors. In fact, it is not very often that psychoanalysis denies anything which is asserted on the other side. As a rule psychoanalysis merely adds something to such assertions and occasionally it does happen that what had hitherto been overlooked, and was newly added by psychoanalysis, is just the essential thing. The influence on the occurrence of tongue slips of such physiological predispositions as result from slight illness, circulatory disturbances and conditions of fatigue, should be acknowledged without more ado. Daily personal experience can convince you of that. But how little is explained by such an admission! Above all, they are not necessary conditions of the errors. Slips of the tongue are just as possible when one is in perfect health and normal condition. Bodily factors, therefore, have only the value of acting by way of facilitation and encouragement to the peculiar psychic mechanism of a slip of the tongue.

To illustrate this relationship, I once used a simile which I will now repeat because I know of no better one as substitute. Let us suppose that some dark night I go past a lonely spot and am there assaulted by a rascal who takes my watch and purse; and then, since I did not see the face of the robber clearly, I make my complaint at the nearest police station in the following words: "Loneliness and darkness have just robbed me of my valuables." The police commissioner could then say to me: "You seem to hold an unjustifiably extreme mechanistic conception. Let us rather state the case as follows: Under cover of darkness, and favored by the loneliness, an unknown robber seized your valuables. The essential task in your case seems to me to be to discover the robber. Perhaps we can then take his booty from him again."

Such psycho-physiological moments as excitement, absent-mindedness and distracted attention, are obviously of small assistance to us for the purpose of explanation. They are mere phrases, screens behind which we will not be deterred from looking. The question is rather what in such cases has caused the excitement, the particular diversion of attention. The influence of syllable sounds, word resemblances and the customary associations which words arouse should also be recognized as having significance. They facilitate the tongue slip by pointing the path which it can take. But if I have a path before me, does that fact as a matter of course determine that I will follow it? After all, I must have a stimulus to make me decide for it, and, in addition, a force which carries me forward on this path. These sound and word relationships therefore serve also only to facilitate the tongue slip, just as the bodily dispositions facilitate them; they cannot give the explanation for the word itself. Just consider, for example, the fact that in an enormously large number of cases, my lecturing is not disturbed by the fact that the words which I use recall others by their sound resemblance, that they are intimately associated with their opposites, or arouse common associations. We might add here the observation of the philosopher Wundt, that slips of the tongue occur when, in consequence of bodily fatigue, the tendency to association gains the upper hand over the intended speech. This would sound very plausible if it were not contradicted by experiences which proved that from one series of cases of tongue-slips bodily stimuli were absent, and from another, the association stimuli were absent.

However, your next question is one of particular interest to me, namely: in what way can one establish the existence of the two mutually antagonistic tendencies? You probably do not suspect how significant this question is. It is true, is it not, that one of the two tendencies, the tendency which suffers the interference, is always unmistakable? The person who commits the error is aware of it and acknowledges it. It is the other tendency, what we call the interfering tendency, which causes doubt and hesitation. Now we have already learned, and you have surely not forgotten, that these tendencies are, in a series of cases, equally plain. That is indicated by the effect of the slip, if only we have the courage to let this effect be valid in itself. The president who said the opposite of what he meant to say made it clear that he wanted to open the meeting, but equally clear that he would also have liked to terminate it. Here the meaning is so plain that there is nothing left to be interpreted. But the other cases in which the interfering tendency merely distorts the original, without bringing itself to full expression—how can one guess the interfering meaning from the distortion?

By a very sure and simple method, in the first series of cases, namely, by the same method by which one establishes the existence of the meaning interfered with. The latter is immediately supplied by the speaker, who instantly adds the originally intended expression. "It may *stake*—no, it may *take* another month." Now we likewise ask him to express the interfering meaning; we ask him: "Now, why did you first say *stake*?" He answers, "I meant to say—'This is a *sorry* business.'" And in the other case of the tongue slip—*re-filed*—the subject also affirms that he meant to say "It is a *fil-thy* business," but then moderated his expression and turned it into something else. Thus the discovery of the interfering meaning was here as successful as the discovery of the one interfered with. Nor did I unintentionally select as examples cases which were neither related nor explained by me or by a supporter of my theories. Yet a certain investigation was necessary in both cases in order to obtain the solution. One had to ask the speaker why he made this slip, what he had to say about it. Otherwise he might perhaps have passed it by without seeking to explain it. When questioned, however, he furnished the explanation by means of the first thing that came to his mind. And now you see, ladies and gentlemen, that this slight investigation and its consequence are already a psychoanalysis, and the prototype of every psychoanalytic investigation which we shall conduct more extensively at a later time.

Now, am I unduly suspicious if I suspect that at the same moment in which psychoanalysis emerges before you, your resistance to psychoanalysis also raises its head? Are you not anxious to raise the objection that the information given by the subject we questioned, and who committed the slip, is not proof sufficient? He naturally has the desire, you say, to meet the challenge, to explain the slip, and hence he says the first thing he can think of if it seems relevant. But that, you say, is no proof that this is really the way the slip happened. It might be so, but it might just as well be otherwise, you say. Something else might have occurred to him which might have fitted the case just as well and better.

It is remarkable how little respect, at bottom, you have for a psychic fact! Imagine that someone has decided to undertake the chemical analysis of a certain substance, and has secured a sample of the substance, of a certain weight—so and so many milligrams. From this weighed sample certain definite conclusions can be drawn. Do you think it would ever occur to a chemist to discredit these conclusions by the argument that the isolated substance might have had some other weight? Everyone yields to the fact that it was just this weight and no other, and confidently builds his further conclusions upon that fact. But when you are confronted by the psychic fact that the subject, when questioned, had a certain idea, you will not accept that as valid, but say some other idea might just as easily have occurred to him! The trouble is that you believe in the illusion of psychic freedom and will not give it up. I regret that on this point I find myself in complete opposition to your views.

Now you will relinquish this point only to take up your resistance at another place. You will continue, "We understand that it is the peculiar technique of psychoanalysis that the solution of its problems is discovered by the analyzed subject himself. Let us take another example, that in which the speaker calls upon the assembly 'to *hiccough* the health of their chief.' The interfering idea in this case, you say, is the insult. It is that which is the antagonist of the expression of conferring an honor. But that is mere interpretation on your part, based on observations extraneous to the slip. If in this case you question the originator of the slip, he will not affirm that he intended an insult, on the contrary, he will deny it energetically. Why do you not give up your unverifiable interpretation in the face of this plain objection?"

Yes, this time you struck a hard problem. I can imagine the unknown speaker. He is probably an assistant to the guest of honor, perhaps already a minor official, a young man with the brightest prospects. I will press him as to whether he did not after all feel conscious of something which may have worked in opposition to the demand that he do honor to the chief. What a fine success I'll have! He becomes impatient and suddenly bursts out on me, "Look here, you'd better stop this cross-examination, or I'll get unpleasant. Why, you'll spoil my whole career with your suspicions. I simply said '*auf*-gestossen' instead of '*an*-gestossen,' because I'd already said '*auf*' twice in the same sentence. It's the thing that Meringer calls a perservation, and there's no other meaning that you can twist out of it. Do you understand me? That's all." H'm, this is a surprising reaction, a really energetic denial. I see that there is nothing more to be obtained from the young man, but I also remark to myself that he betrays a strong personal interest in having his slip mean nothing. Perhaps you, too, agree that it is not right for him immediately to become so rude over a purely theoretical investigation, but, you will conclude, he really must know what he did and did not mean to say.

Really? Perhaps that's open to question nevertheless.

But now you think you have me. "So that is your technique," I hear you say. "When the person who has committed a slip gives an explanation which fits your theory, then you declare him the final authority on the subject. 'He says so himself!' But if what he says does not fit into your scheme, then you suddenly assert that what he says does not count, that one need not believe him."

Yet that is certainly true. I can give you a similar case in which the procedure is apparently just as monstrous. When a defendant confesses to a deed, the judge believes his confession. But if he denies it, the judge does not believe him. Were it otherwise, there would be no way to administer the law, and despite occasional miscarriages you must acknowledge the value of this system.

Well, are you then the judge, and is the person who committed the slip a defendant before you? Is a slip of the tongue a crime?

Perhaps we need not even decline this comparison. But just see to what far-reaching differences we have come by penetrating somewhat into the seemingly harmless problems of the psychology of errors, differences which at this stage we do not at all know how to reconcile. I offer you a preliminary compromise on the basis of the analogy of the judge and the defendant. You will grant me that the meaning of an error admits of no doubt when the subject under analysis acknowledges it himself. I in turn will admit that a direct proof for the suspected meaning cannot be obtained if the subject denies us the information; and, of course, that is also the case when the subject is not present to give us the information. We are, then, as in the case of the legal procedure, dependent on circumstances which make a decision at one time seem more, and at another time, less probable to us. At law, one has to declare a defendant guilty on circumstantial evidence for practical reasons. We see no such necessity; but neither are we forced to forego the use of these circumstances. It would be a mistake to believe that a science consists of nothing but conclusively proved theorems, and any such demand would be unjust. Only a person with a mania for authority, a person who must replace his religious catechism with some other, even though it be scientific, would make such a demand. Science has but few apodeictic precepts in its catechism; it consists chiefly of assertions which it has developed to certain degrees of probability. It is actually a symptom of scientific thinking if one is content with these approximations of certainty and is able to carry on constructive work despite the lack of the final confirmation.

But where do we get the facts for our interpretations, the circumstances for our proof, when the further remarks of the subject under analysis do not themselves elucidate the meaning of the error? From many sources. First of all, from the analogy with phenomena extraneous to the psychology of errors; as, for example, when we assert that the distortion of a name as a slip of the tongue has the same insulting significance as an intentional name distortion. We get them also from the psychic situation in which the error occurred, from our knowledge of the character of the person who committed the error, from the impressions which that person received before making the error, and to which he may possibly have reacted with this error. As a rule, what happens is that we find the meaning of the error according to general principles. It is then only a conjecture, a suggestion as to what the meaning may be, and we then obtain our proof from examination of the psychic situation. Sometimes, too, it happens that we have to wait for subsequent developments, which have announced themselves, as it were, through the error, in order to find our conjecture verified.

I cannot easily give you proof of this if I have to limit myself to the field of tongue slips, although even here there are a few good examples. The young man who wished to "*inscort*" the lady is certainly shy; the lady whose husband may eat and drink whatever *she* wants I know to be one of those energetic women who know how to rule in the home. Or take the following case: At a general meeting of the Concordia Club, a young member delivers a vehement speech in opposition, in the course of which he addresses the officers of the society as: "Fellow committee lenders." We will conjecture that some conflicting idea militated in him against his opposition, an idea which was in some way based on a connection with money lending. As a matter of fact, we learn from our informant that the speaker was in constant money difficulties, and had attempted to raise a loan. As a conflicting idea, therefore, we may safely interpolate the idea, "Be more moderate in your opposition, these are the same people who are to grant you the loan."

But I can give you a wide selection of such circumstantial proof if I delve into the wide field of other kinds of error.

If anyone forgets an otherwise familiar proper name, or has difficulty in retaining it in his memory despite all efforts, then the conclusion lies close at hand, that he has something against the bearer of this name and does not like to think of him. Consider in this connection the following revelation of the psychic situation in which this error occurs:

"A Mr. Y. fell in love, without reciprocation, with a lady who soon after married a Mr. X. In spite of the fact that Mr. Y. has known Mr. X. a long time, and even has business relations with him, he forgets his name over and over again, so that he found it necessary on several occasions to ask other people the man's name when he wanted to write to Mr. X."[12]

Mr. Y. obviously does not want to have his fortunate rival in mind under any condition. "Let him never be thought of."

Another example: A lady makes inquiries at her doctor's concerning a mutual acquaintance, but speaks of her by her maiden name. She has forgotten her married name. She admits that she was much displeased by the marriage, and could not stand this friend's husband.[13]

Later we shall have much to say in other relations about the matter of forgetting names. At present we are predominantly interested in the psychic situation in which the lapse of memory occurs.

The forgetting of projects can quite commonly be traced to an antagonistic current which does not wish to carry out the project. We psychoanalysts are not alone in holding this view, but this is the general conception to which all persons subscribe the daily affairs, and which they first deny in theory. The patron who makes apologies to his protegé, saying that he has forgotten his requests, has not squared himself with his protegé. The protegé immediately thinks: "There's nothing to that; he did promise but he really doesn't want to do it." Hence, daily life also proscribes forgetting, in certain connections, and the difference between the popular and the psychoanalytic conception of these errors appears to be removed. Imagine a housekeeper who receives her guest with the words: "What, you come to-day? Why, I had totally forgotten that I had invited you for to-day"; or the young man who might tell his sweetheart that he had forgotten to keep the rendezvous which they planned. He is sure not to admit it, it were better for him to invent the most improbable excuses on the spur of the moment, hindrances which prevented him from coming at that time, and which made it impossible for him to communicate the situation to her. We all know that in military matters the excuse of having forgotten something is useless, that it protects one from no punishment; and we must consider this attitude justified. Here we suddenly find everyone agreed that a certain error is significant, and everyone agrees what its meaning is. Why are they not consistent enough to extend this insight to the other errors, and fully to acknowledge them? Of course, there is also an answer to this.

If the meaning of this forgetting of projects leaves room for so little doubt among laymen, you will be less surprised to find that poets make use of these errors in the same sense. Those of you who have seen or read Shaw's *Caesar and Cleopatra* will recall that Caesar, when departing in the last scene, is pursued by the idea that there was something more he intended to do, but that he had forgotten it. Finally he discovers what it is: to take leave of Cleopatra. This small device of the author is meant to ascribe to the great Caesar a superiority which he did not possess, and to which he did not at all aspire. You can learn from historical sources that Caesar had Cleopatra follow him to Rome, and that she was staying there with her little Caesarion when Caesar was murdered, whereupon she fled the city.

The cases of forgetting projects are as a rule so clear that they are of little use for our purpose, i.e., discovering in the psychic situation circumstantial evidence of the meaning ofthe error. Let us, therefore, turn to a particularly ambiguous and untransparent error, that of losing and mislaying objects. That we ourselves should have a purpose in losing an object, an accident frequently so painful, will certainly seem incredible to you. But there are many instances similar to the following: A young man loses the pencil which he had liked very much. The day before he had received a letter from his brother-in-law, which concluded with the words, "For the present I have neither the inclination nor the time to be a party to your frivolity and your idleness."[14] It so happened that the pencil had been a present from this brother-in-law. Without this coincidence we could not, of course, assert that the loss involved any intention to get rid of the gift. Similar cases are numerous. Persons lose objects when they have fallen out with the donors, and no longer wish to be reminded of them. Or again, objects may be lost if one no longer likes the things themselves, and wants to supply oneself with a pretext for substituting other and better things in their stead. Letting a thing fall and break naturally shows the same intention toward that object. Can one consider it accidental when a school child just before his birthday loses, ruins or breaks his belongings, for example his school bag or his watch?

He who has frequently experienced the annoyance of not being able to find something which he has himself put away, will also be unwilling to believe there was any intent behind the loss. And yet the examples are not at all rare in which the attendant circumstances of the mislaying point to a tendency temporarily or permanently to get rid of the object. Perhaps the most beautiful example of this sort is the following: A young man tells me: "A few years ago a misunderstanding arose in my married life. I felt my wife was too cool and even though I willingly acknowledged her excellent qualities, we lived without any tenderness between us. One day she brought me a book which she had thought might interest me. I thanked her for this attention, promised to read the book, put it in a handy place, and couldn't find it again. Several months passed thus, during which I occasionally remembered this mislaid book and tried in vain to find it. About half a year later my beloved mother, who lived at a distance from us, fell ill. My wife left the house in order to nurse her mother-in-law. The condition of the patient became serious, and gave my wife an opportunity of showing her best side. One evening I came home filled with enthusiasm and gratitude toward my wife. I approached my writing desk, opened a certain drawer with no definite intention but as if with somnambulistic certainty, and the first thing I found is the book so long mislaid."

With the cessation of the motive, the inability to find the mislaid object also came to an end.

Ladies and gentlemen, I could increase this collection of examples indefinitely. But I do not wish to do so here. In my *Psychopathology of Everyday Life* (first published in 1901), you will find only too many instances for the study of errors.[15]

All these examples demonstrate the same thing repeatedly: namely, they make it seem probable that errors have a meaning, and show how one may guess or establish that meaning from the attendant circumstances. I limit myself to-day because we have confined ourselves to the purpose of profiting in the preparation for psychoanalysis from the study of these phenomena. I must, however, still go into two additional groups of observations, into the accumulated and combined errors and into the confirmation of our interpretations by means of subsequent developments.

The accumulated and combined errors are surely the fine flower of their species. If we were interested only in proving that errors may have a meaning, we would limit ourselves to the accumulated and combined errors in the first place, for here the meaning is unmistakable, even to the dullest intelligence, and can force conviction upon the most critical judgment. The accumulation of manifestations betrays a stubbornness such as could never come about by accident, but which fits closely the idea of design. Finally, the interchange of certain kinds of error with each other shows us what is the important and essential element of the error, not its form or the means of which it avails itself, but the purpose which it serves and which is to be achieved by the most various paths. Thus I will give you a case of repeated forgetting. Jones recounts that he once allowed a letter to lie on his writing desk several days for reasons quite unknown. Finally he made up his mind to mail it; but it was returned from the dead letter office, for he had forgotten to address it. After he had addressed it he took it to the post office, but this time without a stamp. At this point he finally had to admit to himself his aversion against sending the letter at all.

In another case a mistake is combined with mislaying an object. A lady is traveling to Rome with her brother-in-law, a famous artist. The visitor is much fêted by the Germans living in Rome, and receives as a gift, among other things, a gold medal of ancient origin. The lady is vexed by the fact that her brother-in-law does not sufficiently appreciate the beautiful object. After she leaves her sister and reaches her home, she discovers when unpacking that she has brought with her—how, she does not know—the medal. She immediately informs her brother-in-law of this fact by letter, and gives him notice that she will send the medal back to Rome the next day. But on the following day, the medal has been so cleverly mislaid that it can neither be found nor sent, and at this point it begins to dawn upon the lady that her "absent-mindedness" means, namely, that she wants to keep the object for herself.[16]

I have already given you an example of a combination of forgetfulness and error in which someone first forgot a rendezvous and then, with the firm intention of not forgetting it a second time, appeared at the wrong hour. A quite analogous case was told me from his own experience, by a friend who pursues literary interests in addition to his scientific ones. He said: "A few years ago I accepted the election to the board of a certain literary society, because I hoped that the society could at some time be of use to me in helping obtain the production of my drama, and, despite my lack of interest, I took part in the meetings every Friday. A few months ago I received the assurance of a production in the theatre in F., and since that time it happens regularly that I forget the meetings of that society. When I read your article on these things, I was ashamed of my forgetfulness, reproached myself with the meanness of staying away now that I no longer need these people and determined to be sure not to forget next Friday. I kept reminding myself of this resolution until I carried it out and stood before the door of the meeting room. To my astonishment, it was closed, the meeting was already over; for I had mistaken the day. It was already Saturday."

It would be tempting enough to collect similar observations, but I will go no further; I will let you glance instead upon those cases in which our interpretation has to wait for its proof upon future developments.

The chief condition of these cases is conceivably that the existing psychic situation is unknown to us or inaccessible to our inquiries. At that time our interpretation has only the value of a conjecture to which we ourselves do not wish to grant too much weight. Later, however, something happens which shows us how justified was our interpretation even at that time. I was once the guest of a young married couple and heard the young wife laughingly tell of a recent experience, of how on the day after her return from her honeymoon she had hunted up her unmarried sister again in order to go shopping with her, as in former times, while her husband went to his business. Suddenly she noticed a gentleman on the other side of the street, and she nudged her sister, saying, "Why look, there goes Mr. K." She had forgotten that this gentleman was her husband of some weeks' standing. I shuddered at this tale but did not dare to draw the inference. The little anecdote did not occur to me again until a year later, after this marriage had come to a most unhappy end.

A. Maeder tells of a lady who, the day before her wedding, forgot to try on her wedding dress and to the despair of the dressmaker only remembered it later in the evening. He adds in connection with this forgetfulness the fact that she divorced her husband soon after. I know a lady now divorced from her husband, who, in managing her fortune, frequently signed documents with her maiden name, and this many years before she really resumed it. I know of other women who lost their wedding rings on their honeymoon and also know that the course of the marriage gave a meaning to this accident. And now one more striking example with a better termination. It is said that the marriage of a famous German chemist did not take place because he forgot the hour of the wedding, and instead of going to the church went to the laboratory. He was wise enough to rest satisfied with this one attempt, and died unmarried at a ripe old age.

Perhaps the idea has also come to you that in these cases mistakes have taken the place of the *Omina* or omens of the ancients. Some of the *Omina* really were nothing more than mistakes; for example, when a person stumbled or fell down. Others, to be sure, bore the characteristics of objective occurrences rather than that of subjective acts. But you would not believe how difficult it sometimes is to decide in a specific instance whether the act belongs to the one or the other group. It so frequently knows how to masquerade as a passive experience.

Everyone of us who can look back over a longer or shorter life experience will probably say that he might have spared himself many disappointments and painful surprises if he had found the courage and decision to interpret as omens the little mistakes which he made in his intercourse with people, and to consider them as indications of the intentions which were still being kept secret. As a rule, one does not dare do this. One would feel as though he were again becoming superstitious via a detour through science. But not all omens come true, and you will understand from our theories that they need not all come true.

WE may certainly put it down as the conclusion of our labors up to this point that errors have a meaning, and we may make this conclusion the basis of our further investigations. Let me stress the fact once more that we do not assert—and for our purposes need not assert—that every single mistake which occurs is meaningful, although I consider that probable. It will suffice us if we prove the presence of such a meaning with relative frequency in the various forms of errors. These various forms, by the way, behave differently in this respect. In the cases of tongue slips, pen slips, etc., the occurrences may take place on a purely physiological basis. In the group based on forgetfulness (forgetting names or projects, mislaying objects, etc.) I cannot believe in such a basis. There does very probably exist a type of case in which the loss of objects should be recognized as unintentional. Of the mistakes which occur in daily life, only a certain portion can in any way be brought within our conception. You must keep this limitation in mind when we start henceforth from the assumption that mistakes are psychic acts and arise through the mutual interference of two intentions.

Herein we have the first result of psychoanalysis. Psychology hitherto knew nothing of the occurrence of such interferences and the possibility that they might have such manifestations as a consequence. We have widened the province of the world of psychic phenomena quite considerably, and have brought into the province of psychology phenomena which formerly were not attributed to it.

Let us tarry a moment longer over the assertion that errors are psychic acts. Does such an assertion contain more than the former declaration that they have a meaning? I do not believe so. On the contrary, it is rather more indefinite and open to greater misunderstanding. Everything which can be observed about the psychic life will on occasion be designated as a psychic phenomenon. But it will depend on whether the specific psychic manifestations resulted directly from bodily, organic, material influences, in which case their investigation will not fall within the province of psychology, or whether it was more immediately the result of other psychic occurrences back of which, somewhere, the series of organic influences then begins. We have the latter condition of affairs before us when we designate a phenomenon as a psychic manifestation, and for that reason it is more expedient to put our assertion in this form: the phenomena are meaningful; they have a meaning. By "meaning" we understand significance, purpose, tendency and position in a sequence of psychic relations.

There are a number of other occurrences which are very closely related to errors, but which this particular name no longer fits. We call them *accidental and symptomatic* acts. They also have the appearance of being unmotivated, the appearance of insignificance and unimportance, but in addition, and more plainly, of superfluity. They are differentiated from errors by the absence of another intention with which they collide and by which they are disturbed. On the other side they pass over without a definite boundary line into the gestures and movements which we count among expressions of the emotions. Among these accidental acts belong all those apparently playful, apparently purposeless performances in connection with our clothing, parts of our body, objects within reach, as well as the omission of such performances, and the melodies which we hum to ourselves. I venture the assertion that all these phenomena are meaningful and capable of interpretation in the same way as are the errors, that they are small manifestations of other more important psychic processes, valid psychic acts. But I do not intend to linger over this new enlargement of the province of psychic phenomena, but rather to return to the topic of errors, in the consideration of which the important psychoanalytic inquiries can be worked out with far greater clarity.

The most interesting questions which we formulated while considering errors, and which we have not yet answered, are, I presume, the following: We said that the errors are the result of the mutual interference of two different intentions, of which the one can be called the intention interfered with, and the other the interfering intention. The intentions interfered with give rise to no further questions, but concerning the others we want to know, firstly, what kind of intentions are these which arise as disturbers of others, and secondly, in what proportions are the interfering related to the interfered?

Will you permit me again to take the slip of the tongue as representative of the whole species and allow me to answer the second question before the first?

The interfering intention in the tongue slip may stand in a significant relation to the intention interfered with, and then the former contains a contradiction of the latter, correcting or supplementing it. Or, to take a less intelligible and more interesting case, the interfering intention has nothing to do with the intention interfered with.

Proofs for the first of the two relations we can find without trouble in the examples which we already know and in others similar to those. In almost all cases of tongue slips where one says the contrary of what he intended, where the interfering intention expresses the antithesis of the intention interfered with, the error is the presentation of the conflict between two irreconcilable strivings. "I declare the meeting opened, but would rather have it closed," is the meaning of the president's slip. A political paper which has been accused of corruptibility, defends itself in an article meant to reach a climax in the words: "Our readers will testify that we have always interceded for the good of all in the most *disinterested*manner." But the editor who had been entrusted with the composition of the defence, wrote, "in the most *interested* manner." That is, he thinks "To be sure, I have to write this way, but I know better." A representative of the people who urges that the Kaiser should be told the truth "*rückhaltlos*," hears an inner voice which is frightened by his boldness, and which through a slip changes the "*rückhaltlos*" into "*rückgratlos*."[17]

In the examples familiar to you, which give the impression of contraction and abbreviation, it is a question of a correction, an addition or continuation by which the second tendency manifests itself together with the first. "Things were revealed, but better say it right out, they were *filthy*, therefore, things were *refiled*."[18] "The people who understand this topic can be counted on the *fingers of one hand*, but no, there is really only *one* who understands it; therefore, counted *on one finger*." Or, "My husband may eat and drink whatever *he*wants. But you know very well that *I* don't permit him to want anything; therefore he may eat and drink whatever *I want*." In all these cases, therefore, the slip arises from the content of the intention itself, or is connected with it.

The other type of relationship between the two interfering intentions seems strange. If the interfering intention has nothing to do with the content of the one interfered with, where then does it come from and how does it happen to make itself manifest as interference just at that point? The observation which alone can furnish an answer here, recognizes the fact that the interference originates in a thought process which has just previously occupied the person in question and which then has that after-effect, irrespective of whether it has already found expression in speech or not. It is therefore really to be designated as perseveration, but not necessarily as the perseveration of spoken words. Here also there is no lack of an associative connection between the interfering and the interfered with, yet it is not given in the content, but artificially restored, often by means of forced connecting links.

Here is a simple example of this, which I myself observed. In our beautiful Dolomites, I meet two Viennese ladies who are gotten up as tourists. I accompany them a short distance and we discuss the pleasures, but also the difficulties of the tourist's mode of life. One lady admits this way of spending the day entails much discomfort. "It is true," she says, "that it is not at all pleasant, when one has tramped all day in the sun, and waist and shirt are soaked through." At this point in this sentence she suddenly has to overcome a slight hesitancy. Then she continues: "But then, when one gets *nach Hose*, and can change...."[19] We did not analyze this slip, but I am sure you can easily understand it. The lady wanted to make the enumeration more complete and to say, "Waist, shirt and drawers." From motives of propriety, the mention of the drawers (Hose) was suppressed, but in the next sentence of quite independent content the unuttered word came to light as a distortion of the similar word, house (Hause).

Now we can turn at last to the long delayed main question, namely, what kind of intentions are these which get themselves expressed in an unusual way as interferences of others, intentions within whose great variety we wish nevertheless to find what is common to them all! If we examine a series of them to this end, we will soon find that they divide themselves into three groups. In the first group belong the cases in which the interfering tendency is known to the speaker, and which, moreover, was felt by him before the slip. Thus, in the case of the slip "*refilled*," the speaker not only admits that he agreed with the judgment "*filthy*," on the incidents in question, but also that he had the intention (which he later abandoned) of giving it verbal expression. A second group is made up of those cases in which the interfering tendency is immediately recognized by the subject as his own, but in which he is ignorant of the fact that the interfering tendency was active in him just before the slip. He therefore accepts our interpretation, yet remains to a certain extent surprised by it. Examples of this situation can perhaps more easily be found among errors other than slips of the tongue. In a third group the interpretation of the interfering intention is energetically denied by the speaker. He not only denies that the interfering tendency was active in him before the slip, but he wants to assert that it was at all times completely alien to him. Will you recall the example of "hiccough," and the absolutely impolite disavowal which I received at the hands of this speaker by my disclosure of the interfering intention. You know that so far we have no unity in our conception of these cases. I pay no attention to the toastmaster's disavowal and hold fast to my interpretation; while you, I am sure, are yet under the influence of his repudiation and are considering whether one ought not to forego the interpretation of such slips, and let them pass as purely physiological acts, incapable of further analysis. I can imagine what it is that frightens you off. My interpretation draws the conclusion that intentions of which he himself knows nothing may manifest themselves in a speaker, and that I can deduce them from the circumstances. You hesitate before so novel a conclusion and one so full of consequences. I understand that, and sympathize with you to that extent. But let us make one thing clear: if you want consistently to carry through the conception of errors which you have derived from so many examples, you must decide to accept the above conclusion, even though it be unpleasant. If you cannot do so, you must give up that understanding of errors which you have so recently won.

Let us tarry a while over the point which unites the three groups, which is common to the three mechanisms of tongue slips. Fortunately, that is unmistakable. In the first two groups the interfering tendency is recognized by the speaker; in the first there is the additional fact that it showed itself immediately before the slip. In both cases, however, *it was suppressed. The speaker had made up his mind not to convert the interfering tendency into speech and then the slip of the tongue occurred; that is to say, the suppressed tendency obtains expression against the speaker's will, in that it changes the expression of the intention which he permits, mixes itself with it or actually puts itself in its place.* This is, then, the mechanism of the tongue slip.

From my point of view, I can also best harmonize the processes of the third group with the mechanism here described. I need only assume that these three groups are differentiated by the different degrees of effectiveness attending the suppression of an intention. In the first group, the intention is present and makes itself perceptible before the utterance of the speaker; not until then does it suffer the suppression for which it indemnifies itself in the slip. In the second group the suppression extends farther. The intention is no longer perceptible before the subject speaks. It is remarkable that the interfering intention is in no way deterred by this from taking part in the causation of the slip. Through this fact, however, the explanation of the procedure in the third group is simplified for us. I shall be so bold as to assume that in the error a tendency can manifest itself which has been suppressed for even a longer time, perhaps a very long time, which does not become perceptible and which, therefore, cannot be directly denied by the speaker. But leave the problem of the third group; from the observation of the other cases, you most draw the conclusion that *the suppression of the existing intention to say something is the indispensable condition of the occurrence of a slip.*

We may now claim that we have made further progress in understanding errors. We know not only that they are psychic acts, in which we can recognize meaning and purpose, and that they arise through the mutual interference of two different intentions, but, in addition, we know that one of these intentions must have undergone a certain suppression in order to be able to manifest itself through interference with the other. The interfering intention must itself first be interfered with before it can become interfering. Naturally, a complete explanation of the phenomena which we call errors is not attained to by this. We immediately see further questions arising, and suspect in general that there will be more occasions for new questions as we progress further. We might, for example, ask why the matter does not proceed much more simply. If there is an existing purpose to suppress a certain tendency instead of giving it expression, then this suppression should be so successful that nothing at all of the latter comes to light; or it could even fail, so that the suppressed tendency attains to full expression. But errors are compromise formations. They mean some success and some failure for each of the two purposes. The endangered intention is neither completely suppressed nor does it, without regard to individual cases, come through wholly intact. We can imagine that special conditions must be existent for the occurrence of such interference or compromise formations, but then we cannot even conjecture what sort they may be. Nor do I believe that we can uncover these unknown circumstances through further penetration into the study of errors. Rather will it be necessary thoroughly to examine other obscure fields of psychic life. Only the analogies which we there encounter can give us the courage to draw those assumptions which are requisite to a more fundamental elucidation of errors. And one thing more. Even working with small signs, as we have constantly been in the habit of doing in this province, brings its dangers with it. There is a mental disease, combined paranoia, in which the utilization of such small signs is practiced without restriction and I naturally would not wish to give it as my opinion that these conclusions, built up on this basis, are correct throughout. We can be protected from such dangers only by the broad basis of our observations, by the repetition of similar impressions from the most varied fields of psychic life.

We will therefore leave the analysis of errors here. But may I remind you of one thing more: keep in mind, as a prototype, the manner in which we have treated these phenomena. You can see from these examples what the purposes of our psychology are. We do not wish merely to describe the phenomena and to classify them, but to comprehend them as signs of a play of forces in the psychic, as expressions of tendencies striving to an end, tendencies which work together or against one another. We seek a dynamic conception of psychic phenomena. The perceived phenomena must, in our conception, give way to those strivings whose existence is only assumed.

Hence we will not go deeper into the problem of errors, but we can still undertake an expedition through the length of this field, in which we will reëncounter things familiar to us, and will come upon the tracks of some that are new. In so doing we will keep to the division which we made in the beginning of our study, of the three groups of tongue slips, with the related forms of pen slips, misreadings, mishearings, forgetfulness with its subdivisions according to the forgotten object (proper names, foreign words, projects, impressions), and the other faults of mistaking, mislaying and losing objects. Errors, in so far as they come into our consideration, are grouped in part with forgetfulness, in part with mistakes.

We have already spoken in such detail of tongue slips, and yet there are still several points to be added. Linked with tongue slips are smaller effective phenomena which are not entirely without interest. No one likes to make a slip of the tongue; often one fails to hear his own slip, though never that of another. Tongue slips are in a certain sense infectious; it is not at all easy to discuss tongue slips without falling into slips of the tongue oneself. The most trifling forms of tongue slips are just the ones which have no particular illumination to throw on the hidden psychic processes, but are nevertheless not difficult to penetrate in their motivation. If, for example, anyone pronounces a long vowel as a short, in consequence of an interference no matter how motivated, he will for that reason soon after lengthen a short vowel and commit a new slip in compensation for the earlier one. The same thing occurs when one has pronounced a double vowel unclearly and hastily; for example, an "eu" or an "oi" as "ei." The speaker tries to correct it by changing a subsequent "ei" or "eu" to "oi." In this conduct the determining factor seems to be a certain consideration for the hearer, who is not to think that it is immaterial to the speaker how he treats his mother tongue. The second, compensating distortion actually has the purpose of making the hearer conscious of the first, and of assuring him that it also did not escape the speaker. The most frequent and most trifling cases of slips consist in the contractions and foresoundings which show themselves in inconspicuous parts of speech. One's tongue slips in a longer speech to such an extent that the last word of the intended speech is said too soon. That gives the impression of a certain impatience to be finished with the sentence and gives proof in general of a certain resistance to communicating this sentence or speech as a whole. Thus we come to borderline cases in which the differences between the psychoanalytic and the common physiological conception of tongue slips are blended. We assume that in these cases there is a tendency which interferes with the intention of the speech. But it can only announce that it is present, and not what its own intention is. The interference which it occasions then follows some sound influences or associative relationship, and may be considered as a distraction of attention from the intended speech. But neither this disturbance of attention nor the associative tendency which has been activated, strikes the essence of the process. This hints, however, at the existence of an intention which interferes with the purposed speech, an intention whose nature cannot (as is possible in all the more pronounced cases of tongue slips) this time be guessed from its effects.

Slips of the pen, to which I now turn, are in agreement with those of the tongue to the extent that we need expect to gain no new points of view from them. Perhaps we will be content with a small gleaning. Those very common little slips of the pen—contractions, anticipations of later words, particularly of the last words—again point to a general distaste for writing, and to an impatience to be done; the pronounced effects of pen slips permit the nature and purpose of the interfering tendency to be recognized. One knows in general that if one finds a slip of the pen in a letter everything was not as usual with the writer. What was the matter one cannot always establish. The pen slip is frequently as little noticed by the person who makes it as the tongue slip. The following observation is striking: There are some persons who have the habit of always rereading a letter they have written before sending it. Others do not do so. But if the latter make an exception and reread the letter, they always have the opportunity of finding and correcting a conspicuous pen slip. How can that be explained? This looks as if these persons knew that they had made a slip of the pen while writing the letter. Shall we really believe that such is the case?

There is an interesting problem linked with the practical significance of the pen slip. You may recall the case of the murderer H., who made a practice of obtaining cultures of the most dangerous disease germs from scientific institutions, by pretending to be a bacteriologist, and who used these cultures to get his close relatives out of the way in this most modern fashion. This man once complained to the authorities of such an institution about the ineffectiveness of the culture which had been sent to him, but committed a pen slip and instead of the words, "in my attempts on mice and guinea pigs," was plainly written, "in my attempts on people."[20] This slip even attracted the attention of the doctors at the institution, but so far as I know, they drew no conclusion from it. Now what do you think? Might not the doctors better have accepted the slip as a confession and instituted an investigation through which the murderer's handiwork would have been blocked in time? In this case was not ignorance of our conception of errors to blame for an omission of practical importance? Well, I am inclined to think that such a slip would surely seem very suspicious to me, but a fact of great importance stands in the way of its utilization as a confession. The thing is not so simple. The pen slip is surely an indication, but by itself it would not have been sufficient to instigate an investigation. That the man is preoccupied with the thought of infecting human beings, the slip certainly does betray, but it does not make it possible to decide whether this thought has the value of a clear plan of injury or merely of a phantasy having no practical consequence. It is even possible that the person who made such a slip will deny this phantasy with the best subjective justification and will reject it as something entirely alien to him. Later, when we give our attention to the difference between psychic and material reality, you will understand these possibilities even better. Yet this is again a case in which an error later attained unsuspected significance.

In misreading, we encounter a psychic situation which is clearly differentiated from that of the tongue slips or pen slips. The one of the two rival tendencies is here replaced by a sensory stimulus and perhaps for that reason is less resistant. What one is reading is not a production of one's own psychic activity, as is something which one intends to write. In a large majority of cases, therefore, the misreading consists in a complete substitution. One substitutes another word for the word to be read, and there need be no connection in meaning between the text and the product of the misreading. In general, the slip is based upon a word resemblance. Lichtenberg's example of reading *"Agamemnon"* for *"angenommen"*[21] is the best of this group. If one wishes to discover the interfering tendency which causes the misreading, one may completely ignore the misread text and can begin the analytic investigation with the two questions: What is the first idea that occurs in free association to the product of the misreading, and, in what situation did the misreading occur? Now and then a knowledge of the latter suffices by itself to explain the misreading. Take, for example, the individual who, distressed by certain needs, wanders about in a strange city and reads the word *"Closethaus"* on a large sign on the first floor of a house. He has just time to be surprised at the fact that the sign has been nailed so high up when he discovers that, accurately observed, the sign reads *"Corset-haus."* In other cases the misreadings which are independent of the text require a penetrating analysis which cannot be accomplished without practice and confidence in the psychoanalytic technique. But generally it is not a matter of much difficulty to obtain the elucidation of a misreading. The substituted word, as in the example, *"Agamemnon,"* betrays without more ado the thought sequence from which the interference results. In war times, for instance, it is very common for one to read into everything which contains a similar word structure, the names of the cities, generals and military expressions which are constantly buzzing around us. In this way, whatever interests and preoccupies one puts itself in the place of that which is foreign or uninteresting. The after-effects of thoughts blur the new perceptions.

There are other types of misreadings, in which the text itself arouses the disturbing tendency, by means of which it is then most often changed into its opposite. One reads something which is undesired; analysis then convinces one that an intensive wish to reject what has been read should be made responsible for the alteration.

In the first mentioned and more frequent cases of misreading, two factors are neglected to which we gave an important role in the mechanism of errors: the conflict of two tendencies and the suppression of one which then indemnifies itself by producing the error. Not that anything like the opposite occurs in misreading, but the importunity of the idea content which leads to misreading is nevertheless much more conspicuous than the suppression to which the latter may previously have been subjected. Just these two factors are most tangibly apparent in the various situations of errors of forgetfulness.

Forgetting plans is actually uniform in meaning; its interpretation is, as we have heard, not denied even by the layman. The tendency interfering with the plan is always an antithetical intention, an unwillingness concerning which we need only discover why it does not come to expression in a different and less disguised manner. But the existence of this unwillingness is not to be doubted. Sometimes it is possible even to guess something of the motives which make it necessary for this unwillingness to disguise itself, and it always achieves its purpose by the error resulting from the concealment, while its rejection would be certain were it to present itself as open contradiction. If an important change in the psychic situation occurs between the formulation of the plan and its execution, in consequence of which the execution of the plan does not come into question, then the fact that the plan was forgotten is no longer in the class of errors. One is no longer surprised at it, and one understands that it would have been superfluous to have remembered the plan; it was then permanently or temporarily effaced. Forgetting a plan can be called an error only when we have no reason to believe there was such an interruption.

The cases of forgetting plans are in general so uniform and transparent that they do not interest us in our investigation. There are two points, however, from which we can learn something new. We have said that forgetting, that is, the non-execution of a plan, points to an antipathy toward it. This certainly holds, but, according to the results of our investigations, the antipathy may be of two sorts, direct and indirect. What is meant by the latter can best be explained by one or two examples. If a patron forgets to say a good word for his protegé to a third person, it may be because the patron is not really very much interested in the protegé, therefore, has no great inclination to commend him. It is, at any rate, in this sense that the protegé will construe his patron's forgetfulness. But the matter may be more complicated. The patron's antipathy to the execution of the plan may originate in another quarter and fasten upon quite a different point. It need not have anything to do with the protegé, but may be directed toward the third person to whom the good word was to have been said. Thus, you see what doubts here confront the practical application of our interpretation. The protegé, despite a correct interpretation of the forgetfulness, stands in danger of becoming too suspicious, and of doing his patron a grave injustice. Or, if an individual forgets a rendezvous which he has made, and which he had resolved to keep, the most frequent basis will certainly be the direct aversion to encountering this person. But analysis might here supply the information that the interfering intention was not directed against that person, but against the place in which they were to have met, and which was avoided because of a painful memory associated with it. Or, if one forgets to mail a letter, the counter-intention may be directed against the content of that letter, yet this does not in any way exclude the possibility that the letter is harmless in itself, and only subject to the counter-intention because something about it reminds the writer of another letter written previously, which, in fact, did afford a basis for the antipathy. One can say in such a case that the antipathy has here transferred itself from that former letter where it was justified to the present one in which it really has no meaning. Thus you see that one must always exercise restraint and caution in the application of interpretations, even though the interpretations are justified. That which is psychologically equivalent may nevertheless in practice be very ambiguous.

Phenomena such as these will seem very unusual to you. Perhaps you are inclined to assume that the "indirect" antipathy is enough to characterize the incident as pathological. Yet I can assure you that it also occurs in a normal and healthy setting. I am in no way willing to admit the unreliability of our analytic interpretation. After all, the above-discussed ambiguity of plan-forgetting exists only so long as we have not attempted an analysis of the case, and are interpreting it only on the basis of our general suppositions. When we analyze the person in question, we discover with sufficient certainty in each case whether or not it is a direct antipathy, or what its origin is otherwise.

A second point is the following: when we find in a large majority of cases that the forgetting of a plan goes back to an antipathy, we gain courage to extend this solution to another series of cases in which the analyzed person does not confirm, but denies, the antipathy which we inferred. Take as an example the exceedingly frequent incidents of forgetting to return books which one has borrowed, or forgetting to pay one's bills or debts. We will be so bold as to accuse the individual in question of intending to keep the books and not to pay the debts, while he will deny such an intention but will not be in a position to give us any other explanation of his conduct. Thereupon we insist that he has the intention, only he knows nothing about it; all we need for our inference is to have the intention betray itself through the effect of the forgetfulness. The subject may then repeat that he had merely forgotten it. You now recognize the situation as one in which we once before found ourselves. If we wish to be consistent in our interpretation, an interpretation which has been proved as manifold as it is justified, we will be unavoidably forced to the conclusion that there are tendencies in a human being which can become effective without his being conscious of them. By so doing, however, we place ourselves in opposition to all the views which prevail in daily life and in psychology.

Forgetting proper names and foreign names as well as foreign words can be traced in the same manner to a counter-intention which aims either directly or indirectly at the name in question. I have already given you an example of such direct antipathy. The indirect causation, however, is particularly frequent and generally necessitates careful analysis for its determination. Thus, for example, in war times which force us to sacrifice so many of our former inclinations, the ability to recall proper names also suffers severely in consequence of the most peculiar connections. A short time ago it happened that I could not reproduce the name of that harmless Moravian city of Bisenz, and analysis showed that no direct dislike was to blame, but rather the sound resemblance to the name of the Bisenzi palace in Orrieto, in which I used to wish I might live. As a motive for the antagonism to remembering the name, we here encounter for the first time a principle which will later disclose to us its whole tremendous significance in the causation of neurotic symptoms, viz., the aversion on the part of the memory to remembering anything which is connected with unpleasant experience and which would revive this unpleasantness by a reproduction. This intention of avoiding unpleasantness in recollections of other psychic acts, the psychic flight from unpleasantness, we may recognize as the ultimate effective motive not only for the forgetting of names, but also for many other errors, such as omissions of action, etc.

Forgetting names does, however, seem to be especially facilitated psycho-physiologically and therefore also occurs in cases in which the interference of an unpleasantness-motive cannot be established. If anyone once has a tendency to forget names, you can establish by analytical investigation that he not only loses names because he himself does not like them, or because they remind him of something he does not like, but also because the same name in his mind belongs to another chain of associations, with which he has more intimate relations. The name is anchored there, as it were, and denied to the other associations activated at the moment. If you will recall the tricks of mnemonic technique you will ascertain with some surprise that one forgets names in consequence of the same associations which one otherwise purposely forms in order to save them from being forgotten. The most conspicuous example of this is afforded by proper names of persons, which conceivably enough must have very different psychic values for different people. For example, take a first name, such as Theodore. To one of you it will mean nothing special, to another it means the name of his father, brother, friend, or his own name. Analytic experience will then show you that the first person is not in danger of forgetting that a certain stranger bears this name, while the latter will be constantly inclined to withhold from the stranger this name which seems reserved for intimate relationships. Let us now assume that this associative inhibition can come into contact with the operation of the unpleasantness-principle, and in addition with an indirect mechanism, and you will be in a position to form a correct picture of the complexity of causation of this temporary name-forgetting. An adequate analysis that does justice to the facts, however, will completely disclose these complications.

Forgetting impressions and experiences shows the working of the tendency to keep unpleasantness from recollection much more clearly and conclusively than does the forgetting of names. It does not, of course, belong in its entirety to the category of errors, but only in so far as it seems to us conspicuous and unjustified, measured by the measuring stick of our accustomed conception—thus, for example, where the forgetfulness strikes fresh or important impressions or impressions whose loss tears a hole in the otherwise well-remembered sequence. Why and how it is in general that we forget, particularly why and how we forget experiences which have surely left the deepest impressions, such as the incidents of our first years of childhood, is quite a different problem, in which the defense against unpleasant associations plays a certain role but is far from explaining everything. That unpleasant impressions are easily forgotten is an indubitable fact. Various psychologists have observed it, and the great Darwin was so struck by it that he made the "golden rule" for himself of writing down with particular care observations which seemed unfavorable to his theory, since he had convinced himself that they were just the ones which would not stick in his memory.

Those who hear for the first time of this principle of defense against unpleasant recollections by means of forgetting, seldom fail to raise the objection that they, on the contrary, have had the experience that just the painful is hard to forget, inasmuch as it always comes back to mind to torture the person against his will— as, for example, the recollection of an insult or humiliation. This fact is also correct, but the objection is not valid. It is important that one begin betimes to reckon with the fact that the psychic life is the arena of the struggles and exercises of antagonistic tendencies, or, to express it in non-dynamic terminology, that it consists of contradictions and paired antagonisms. Information concerning one specific tendency is of no avail for the exclusion of its opposite; there is room for both of them. It depends only on how the opposites react upon each other, what effects will proceed from the one and what from the other.

Losing and mislaying objects is of especial interest to us because of the ambiguity and the multiplicity of tendencies in whose services the errors may act. The common element in all cases is this, that one wished to lose something. The reasons and purposes thereof vary. One loses an object when it has become damaged, when one intends to replace it with a better one, when one has ceased to like it, when it came from a person whose relations to one have become strained, or when it was obtained under circumstances of which one no longer wishes to think. The same purpose may be served by letting the object fall, be damaged or broken. In the life of society it is said to have been found that unwelcome and illegitimate children are much more often frail than those born in wedlock. To reach this result we do not need the coarse technique of the so-called angel-maker. A certain remissness in the care of the child is said to suffice amply. In the preservation of objects, the case might easily be the same as with the children.

But things may be singled out for loss without their having forfeited any of their value, namely, when there exists the intention to sacrifice something to fate in order to ward off some other dreaded loss. Such exorcisings of fate are, according to the findings of analysis, still very frequent among us; therefore, the loss of things is often a voluntary sacrifice. In the same way losing may serve the purposes of obstinacy or self-punishment. In short, the more distant motivation of the tendency to get rid of a thing oneself by means of losing it is not overlooked.

Mistakes, like other errors, are often used to fulfill wishes which one ought to deny oneself. The purpose is thus masked as fortunate accident; for instance, one of our friends once took the train to make a call in the suburbs, despite the clearest antipathy to so doing, and then, in changing cars, made the mistake of getting into the train which took him back to the city. Or, if on a trip one absolutely wants to make a longer stay at a half-way station, one is apt to overlook or miss certain connections, so that he is forced to make the desired interruption to the trip. Or, as once happened to a patient of mine whom I had forbidden to call up his fiancée on the telephone, "by mistake" and "absent-mindedly" he asked for a wrong number when he wanted to telephone to me, so that he was suddenly connected with the lady. A pretty example and one of practical significance in making a direct mistake is the observation of an engineer at a preliminary hearing in a damage suit:

"Some time ago I worked with several colleagues in the laboratory of a high school on a series of complicated elasticity experiments, a piece of work which we had undertaken voluntarily but which began to take more time than we had expected. One day as I went into the laboratory with my colleague F., the latter remarked how unpleasant it was to him to lose so much time that day, since he had so much to do at home. I could not help agreeing with him, and remarked half jokingly, alluding to an incident of the previous week: 'Let's hope that the machine gives out again so that we can stop work and go home early.'

"In the division of labor it happened that F. was given the regulation of the valve of the press, that is to say, he was, by means of a cautious opening of the valve, to let the liquid pressure from the accumulator flow slowly into the cylinder of the hydraulic press. The man who was directing the job stood by the manometer (pressure gauge) and when the right pressure had been reached called out in a loud voice: 'Stop.' At this command F. seized the valve and turned with all his might—to the left! (All valves, without exception, close to the right.) Thereby the whole pressure of the accumulator suddenly became effective in the press, a strain for which the connecting pipes are not designed, so that a connecting pipe immediately burst—quite a harmless defect, but one which nevertheless forced us to drop work for the day and go home.

"It is characteristic, by the way, that some time afterward when we were discussing this occurrence, my friend F. had no recollection whatever of my remark, which I could recall with certainty."

From this point you may reach the conjecture that it is not harmless accident which makes the hands of your domestics such dangerous enemies to your household property. But you can also raise the question whether it is always an accident when one damages himself and exposes his own person to danger. There are interests the value of which you will presently be able to test by means of the analysis of observations.

Ladies and gentlemen, this is far from being all that might be said about errors. There is indeed much left to investigate and to discuss. But I am satisfied if, from our investigations to date, your previous views are somewhat shaken and if you have acquired a certain degree of liberality in the acceptance of new ones. For the rest, I must content myself with leaving you face to face with an unclear condition of affairs. We cannot prove all our axioms by the study of errors and, indeed, are by no means solely dependent on this material. The great value of errors for our purpose lies in the fact that they are very frequent phenomena that can easily be observed on oneself and the occurrence of which do not require a pathological condition. I should like to mention just one more of your unanswered questions before concluding: "If, as we have seen in many examples, people come so close to understanding errors and so often act as though they penetrated their meaning, how is it possible that they can so generally consider them accidental, senseless and meaningless, and can so energetically oppose their psychoanalytic elucidation?"

You are right; that is conspicuous and demands an explanation. I shall not give this explanation to you, however, but shall guide you slowly to the connecting links from which the explanation will force itself upon you without any aid from me.

II

THE DREAM

FIFTH LECTURE

THE DREAM

Difficulties and Preliminary Approach

ONE day the discovery was made that the disease symptoms of certain nervous patients have a meaning.[22] Thereupon the psychoanalytic method of therapy was founded. In this treatment it happened that the patients also presented dreams in place of their symptoms. Herewith originated the conjecture that these dreams also have a meaning.

We will not, however, pursue this historical path, but enter upon the opposite one. We wish to discover the meaning of dreams as preparation for the study of the neuroses. This inversion is justified, for the study of dreams is not only the best preparation for that of the neuroses, but the dream itself is also a neurotic symptom, and in fact one which possesses for us the incalculable advantage of occurring in all normals. Indeed, if all human beings were well and would dream, we could gain from their dreams almost all the insight to which the study of the neuroses has led.

Thus it is that the dream becomes the object of psychoanalytic research—again an ordinary, little-considered phenomenon, apparently of no practical value, like the errors with which, indeed, it shares the character of occurring in normals. But otherwise the conditions are rather less favorable for our work. Errors had been neglected only by science, which had paid little attention to them; but at least it was no disgrace to occupy one's self with them. People said there are indeed more important things, but perhaps something may come of it. Preoccupation with the dream, however, is not merely impractical and superfluous, but actually ignominious; it carries the odium of the unscientific, awakens the suspicion of a personal leaning towards mysticism. The idea of a physician busying himself with dreams when even in neuropathology and psychiatry there are matters so much more serious—tumors the size of apples which incapacitate the organ of the psyche, hemorrhages, and chronic inflammations in which one can demonstrate changes in the tissues under the microscope! No, the dream is much too trifling an object, and unworthy of Science.

And besides, it is a condition which in itself defies all the requirements of exact research—in dream investigation one is not even sure of one's object. A delusion, for example, presents itself in clear and definite outlines. "I am the Emperor of China," says the patient aloud. But the dream? It generally cannot be related at all. If anyone relates a dream, has he any guarantee that he has told it correctly, and not changed it during the telling, or invented an addition which was forced by the indefiniteness of his recollection? Most dreams cannot be remembered at all, are forgotten except for small fragments. And upon the interpretation of such material shall a scientific psychology or method of treatment for patients be based?

A certain excess in judgment may make us suspicious. The objections to the dream as an object of research obviously go too far. The question of insignificance we have already had to deal with in discussing errors. We said to ourselves that important matters may manifest themselves through small signs. As concerns the indefiniteness of the dream, it is after all a characteristic like any other. One cannot prescribe the characteristics of an object. Moreover, there are clear and definite dreams. And there are other objects of psychiatric research which suffer from the same trait of indefiniteness, e.g., many compulsion ideas, with which even respectable and esteemed psychiatrists have occupied themselves. I might recall the last case which occurred in my practice. The patient introduced himself to me with the words, "I have a certain feeling as though I had harmed or had wished to harm some living thing—a child?—no, more probably a dog—perhaps pushed it off a bridge—or something else." We can overcome to some degree the difficulty of uncertain recollection in the dream if we determine that exactly what the dreamer tells us is to be taken as his dream, without regard to anything which he has forgotten or may have changed in recollection. And finally, one cannot make so general an assertion as that the dream is an unimportant thing. We know from our own experience that the mood in which one wakes up after a dream may continue throughout the whole day. Cases have been observed by physicians in which a psychosis begins with a dream and holds to a delusion which originated in it. It is related of historical personages that they drew their inspiration for important deeds from dreams. So we may ask whence comes the contempt of scientific circles for the dream?

I think it is the reaction to their over-estimation in former times. Reconstruction of the past is notoriously difficult, but this much we may assume with certainty—if you will permit me the jest—that our ancestors of 3000 years ago and more, dreamed much in the way we do. As far as we know, all ancient peoples attached great importance to dreams and considered them of practical value. They drew omens for the future from dreams, sought premonitions in them. In those days, to the Greeks and all Orientals, a campaign without dream interpreters must have been as impossible as a campaign without an aviation scout to-day. When Alexander the Great undertook his campaign of conquests, the most famous dream interpreters were in attendance. The city of Tyrus, which was then still situated on an island, put up so fierce a resistance that Alexander considered the idea of raising the siege. Then he dreamed one night of a satyr dancing as if in triumph; and when he laid his dream before his interpreters he received the information that the victory over the city had been announced to him. He ordered the attack and took Tyrus. Among the Etruscans and the Romans other methods of discovering the future were in use, but the interpretation of dreams was practical and esteemed during the entire Hellenic-Roman period. Of the literature dealing with the topic at least the chief work has been preserved to us, namely, the book of Artemidoros of Daldis, who is supposed to have lived during the lifetime of the Emperor Hadrian. How it happened subsequently that the art of dream interpretation was lost and the dream fell into discredit, I cannot tell you. Enlightenment cannot have had much part in it, for the Dark Ages faithfully preserved things far more absurd than the ancient dream interpretation. The fact is, the interest in dreams gradually deteriorated into superstition, and could assert itself only among the ignorant. The latest misuse of dream interpretation in our day still tries to discover in dreams the numbers which are going to be drawn in the small lottery. On the other hand, the exact science of to-day has repeatedly dealt with dreams, but always only with the purpose of applying its physiological theories to the dream. By physicians, of course, the dream was considered as a non-psychic act, as the manifestation of somatic irritations in the psychic life. Binz (1876) pronounced the dream "a bodily process, in all cases useless, in many actually pathological, above which the world-soul and immortality are raised as high as the blue ether over the weed-grown sands of the lowest plain." Maury compared it with the irregular twitchings of St. Vitus' Dance in contrast to the co-ordinated movements of the normal person. An old comparison makes the content of the dream analogous to the tones which the "ten fingers of a musically illiterate person would bring forth if they ran over the keys of the instrument."

Interpretation means finding a hidden meaning. There can be no question of interpretation in such an estimation of the dream process. Look up the description of the dream in Wundt, Jodl and other newer philosophers. You will find an enumeration of the deviations of dream life from waking thought, in a sense disparaging to the dream. The description points out the disintegration of association, the suspension of the critical faculty, the elimination of all knowledge, and other signs of diminished activity. The only valuable contribution to the knowledge of the dream which we owe to exact science pertains to the influence of bodily stimuli, operative during sleep, on the content of the dream. There are two thick volumes of experimental researches on dreams by the recently deceased Norwegian author, J. Mourly Vold, (translated into German in 1910 and 1912), which deal almost solely with the consequences of changes in the position of the limbs. They are recommended as the prototype of exact dream research. Now can you imagine what exact science would say if it discovered that we wish to attempt to find the meaning of dreams? It may be it has already said it, but we will not allow ourselves to be frightened off. If errors can have a meaning, the dream can, too, and errors in many cases have a meaning which has escaped exact science. Let us confess to sharing the prejudice of the ancients and the common people, and let us follow in the footsteps of the ancient dream interpreters.

First of all, we must orient ourselves in our task, and take a bird's eye view of our field. What is a dream? It is difficult to say in one sentence. But we do not want to attempt any definition where a reference to the material with which everyone is familiar suffices. Yet we ought to select the essential element of the dream. How can that be found? There are such monstrous differences within the boundary which encloses our province, differences in every direction. The essential thing will very probably be that which we can show to be common to all dreams.

Well, the first thing which is common to all dreams is that we are asleep during their occurrence. The dream is apparently the psychic life during sleep, which has certain resemblances to that of the waking condition, and on the other hand is distinguished from it by important differences. That was noted even in Aristotle's definition. Perhaps there are other connections obtaining between the dream and sleep. One can be awakened by a dream, one frequently has a dream when he wakes spontaneously or is forcibly awakened from sleep. The dream then seems to be an intermediate condition between sleeping and waking. Thus we are referred to the problem of sleep. What, then, is sleep?

That is a physiological or biological problem concerning which there is still much controversy. We can form no decision on the point, but I think we may attempt a psychological characterization of sleep. Sleep is a condition in which I wish to have nothing to do with the external world, and have withdrawn my interest from it. I put myself to sleep by withdrawing myself from the external world and by holding off its stimuli. I also go to sleep when I am fatigued by the external world. Thus, by going to sleep, I say to the external world, "Leave me in peace, for I wish to sleep." Conversely, the child says, "I won't go to bed yet, I am not tired, I want to have some more fun." The biological intention of sleep thus seems to be recuperation; its psychological character, the suspension of interest in the external world. Our relation to the world into which we came so unwillingly, seems to include the fact that we cannot endure it without interruption. For this reason we revert from time to time to the pre-natal existence, that is, to the intra-uterine existence. At least we create for ourselves conditions quite similar to those obtaining at that time—warmth, darkness and the absence of stimuli. Some of us even roll ourselves into tight packages and assume in sleep a posture very similar to the intra-uterine posture. It seems as if the world did not wholly possess us adults, it has only two-thirds of our life, we are still one-third unborn. Each awakening in the morning is then like a new birth. We also speak of the condition after sleep with the words, "I feel as though I had been born anew," by which we probably form a very erroneous idea of the general feeling of the newly born. It may be assumed that the latter, on the contrary, feel very uncomfortable. We also speak of birth as "seeing the light of day." If that be sleep, then the dream is not on its program at all, rather it seems an unwelcome addition. We think, too, that dreamless sleep is the best and only normal sleep. There should be no psychic activity in sleep; if the psyche stirs, then just to that extent have we failed to reduplicate the foetal condition; remainders of psychic activity could not be completely avoided. These remainders are the dream. Then it really does seem that the dream need have no meaning. It was different in the case of errors; they were activities of the waking state. But when I am asleep, have quite suspended psychic activity and have suppressed all but certain of its remainders, then it is by no means inevitable that these remainders have a meaning. In fact, I cannot make use of this meaning, in view of the fact that the rest of my psyche is asleep. This must, of course, be a question only of twitching, like spasmodic reactions, a question only of psychic phenomena such as follow directly upon somatic stimulation. The dream, therefore, appears to be the sleep-disturbing remnant of the psychic activity of waking life, and we may make the resolution promptly to abandon a theme which is so ill-adapted to psychoanalysis.

However, even if the dream is superfluous, it exists nevertheless and we may try to give an account of its existence. Why does not the psyche go to sleep? Probably because there is something which gives it no rest. Stimuli act upon the psyche, and it must react to them. The dream, therefore, is the way in which the psyche reacts to the stimuli acting upon it in the sleeping condition. We note here a point of approach to the understanding of the dream. We can now search through different dreams to discover what are the stimuli which seek to disturb the sleep and which are reacted to with dreams. Thus far we might be said to have discovered the first common element.

Are there other common elements? Yes, it is undeniable that there are, but they are much more difficult to grasp and describe. The psychic processes of sleep, for example, have a very different character from those of waking. One experiences many things in the dream, and believes in them, while one really has experienced nothing but perhaps the one disturbing stimulus. One experiences them predominantly in visual images; feelings may also be interspersed in the dream as well as thoughts; the other senses may also have experiences, but after all the dream experiences are predominantly pictures. A part of the difficulty of dream telling comes from the fact that we have to transpose these pictures into words. "I could draw it," the dreamer says frequently, "but I don't know how to say it." That is not really a case of diminished psychic activity, like that of the feeble-minded in comparison with the highly gifted; it is something qualitatively different, but it is difficult to say wherein the difference lies. G. T. Fechner once hazarded the conjecture that the scene in which dreams are played is a different one from that of the waking perceptual life. To be sure, we do not understand this, do not know what we are to think of it, but the impression of strangeness which most dreams make upon us does really bear this out. The comparison of the dream activity with the effects of a hand untrained in music also fails at this point. The piano, at least, will surely answer with the same tones, even if not with melodies, as soon as by accident one brushes its keys. Let us keep this second common element of all dreams carefully in mind, even though it be not understood.

Are there still further traits in common? I find none, and see only differences everywhere, differences indeed in the apparent length as well as the definiteness of the activities, participation of effects, durability, etc. All this really is not what we might expect of a compulsion-driven, irresistible, convulsive defense against a stimulus. As concerns the dimensions of dreams, there are very short ones which contain only one picture or a few, one thought—yes, even one word only—, others which are uncommonly rich in content, seem to dramatize whole novels and to last very long. There are dreams which are as plain as an experience itself, so plain that we do not recognize them as dreams for a long time after waking; others which are indescribably weak, shadowy and vague; indeed in one and the same dream, the overemphasized and the scarcely comprehensible, indefinite parts may alternate with each other. Dreams may be quite meaningful or at least coherent, yes, even witty, fantastically beautiful. Others, again, are confused, as if feeble-minded, absurd, often actually mad. There are dreams which leave us quite cold, others in which all the effects come to expression—pain deep enough for tears, fear strong enough to waken us, astonishment, delight, etc. Dreams are generally quickly forgotten upon waking, or they may hold over a day to such an extent as to be faintly and incompletely remembered in the evening. Others, for example, the dreams of childhood, are so well preserved that they stay in the memory thirty years later, like fresh experiences. Dreams, like individuals, may appear a single time, and never again, or they may repeat themselves unchanged in the same person, or with small variations. In short, this nightly psychic activity can avail itself of an enormous repertoire, can indeed compass everything which the psychic accomplishes by day, but yet the two are not the same.

One might try to give an account of this many-sidedness of the dream by assuming that it corresponds to different intermediate stages between sleeping and waking, different degrees of incomplete sleep. Yes, but in that case as the psyche nears the waking state, the conviction that it is a dream ought to increase along with the value, content and distinctiveness of the dream product, and it would not happen that immediately beside a distinct and sensible dream fragment a senseless and indistinct one would occur, to be followed again by a goodly piece of work. Surely the psyche could not change its degree of somnolence so quickly. This explanation thus avails us nothing; at any rate, it cannot be accepted offhand.

Let us, for the present, give up the idea of finding the meaning of the dream and try instead to clear a path to a better understanding of the dream by means of the elements common to all dreams. From the relation of dreams to the sleeping condition, we concluded that the dream is the reaction to a sleep-disturbing stimulus. As we have heard, this is the only point upon which exact experimental psychology can come to our assistance; it gives us the information that stimuli applied during sleep appear in the dream. There have been many such investigations carried out, including that of the above mentioned Mourly Vold. Indeed, each of us must at some time have been in a position to confirm this conclusion by means of occasional personal observations. I shall choose certain older experiments for presentation. Maury had such experiments made on his own person. He was allowed to smell cologne while dreaming. He dreamed that he was in Cairo in the shop of Johann Marina Farina, and therewith were linked further extravagant adventures. Or, he was slightly pinched in the nape of the neck; he dreamed of having a mustard plaster applied, and of a doctor who had treated him in childhood. Or, a drop of water was poured on his forehead. He was then in Italy, perspired profusely, and drank the white wine of Orvieto.

What strikes us about these experimentally induced dreams we may perhaps be able to comprehend still more clearly in another series of stimulated dreams. Three dreams have been recounted by a witty observer, Hildebrand, all of them reactions to the sound of the alarm clock:

"I go walking one spring morning and saunter through the green fields to a neighboring village. There I see the inhabitants in gala attire, their hymn books under their arms, going church-ward in great numbers. To be sure, this is Sunday, and the early morning service will soon begin. I decide to attend, but since I am somewhat overheated, decide to cool off in the cemetery surrounding the church. While I am there reading several inscriptions, I hear the bell ringer ascend the tower, and now see the little village church bell which is to give the signal for the beginning of the service. The bell hangs a good bit longer, then it begins to swing, and suddenly its strokes sound clear and penetrating, so clear and penetrating that they make an end of—my sleep. The bell-strokes, however, come from my alarm clock.

"A second combination. It is a clear winter day. The streets are piled high with snow. I agree to go on a sleighing party, but must wait a long time before the announcement comes that the sleigh is at the door. Then follow the preparations for getting in—the fur coat is put on, the footwarmer dragged forth—and finally I am seated in my place. But the departure is still delayed until the reins give the waiting horses the tangible signal. Now they pull; the vigorously shaken bells begin their familiar Janizary music so powerfully that instantly the spider web of the dream is torn. Again it is nothing but the shrill tone of the alarm clock.

"And still a third example. I see a kitchen maid walking along the corridor to the dining room with some dozens of plates piled high. The pillar of porcelain in her arms seems to me in danger of losing its balance. 'Take care!' I warn her. 'The whole load will fall to the ground.' Naturally, the inevitable retort follows: one is used to that, etc., and I still continue to follow the passing figure with apprehensive glances. Sure enough, at the threshold she stumbles—the brittle dishes fall and rattle and crash over the floor in a thousand pieces. But—the endless racket is not, as I soon notice, a real rattling, but really a ringing and with this ringing, as the awakened subject now realizes, the alarm has performed its duty."

These dreams are very pretty, quite meaningful, not at all incoherent, as dreams usually are. We will not object to them on that score. That which is common to them all is that the situation terminates each time in a noise, which one recognizes upon waking up as the sound of the alarm. Thus we see here how a dream originates, but also discover something else. The dream does not recognize the alarm—indeed the alarm does not appear in the dream—the dream replaces the alarm sound with another, it interprets the stimulus which interrupts the sleep, but interprets it each time in a different way. Why? There is no answer to this question, it seems to be something arbitrary. But to understand the dream means to be able to say why it has chosen just this sound and no other for the interpretation of the alarm-clock stimulus. In quite analogous fashion, we must raise the objection to the Maury experiment that we see well enough that the stimulus appears in the dream, but that we do not discover why it appears in just this form; and that the form taken by the dream does not seem to follow from the nature of the sleep-disturbing stimulus. Moreover, in the Maury experiments a mass of other dream material links itself to the direct stimulus product; as, for example, the extravagant adventures in the cologne dream, for which one can give no account.

Now I shall ask you to consider the fact that the waking dreams offer by far the best chances for determining the influence of external sleep-disturbing stimuli. In most of the other cases it will be more difficult. One does not wake up in all dreams, and in the morning, when one remembers the dream of the night, how can one discover the disturbing stimulus which was perhaps in operation at night? I did succeed once in subsequently establishing such a sound stimulus, though naturally only in consequence of special circumstances. I woke up one morning in a place in the Tyrolese Mountains, with the certainty that I had dreamt the Pope had died. I could not explain the dream, but then my wife asked me: "Did you hear the terrible bell ringing that broke out early this morning from all the churches and chapels?" No, I had heard nothing, my sleep is a sound one, but thanks to this information I understood my dream. How often may such stimuli incite the sleeper to dream without his knowing of them afterward? Perhaps often, perhaps infrequently; when the stimulus can no longer be traced, one cannot be convinced of its existence. Even without this fact we have given up evaluating the sleep disturbing stimuli, since we know that they can explain only a little bit of the dream, and not the whole dream reaction.

But we need not give up this whole theory for that reason. In fact, it can be extended. It is clearly immaterial through what cause the sleep was disturbed and the psyche incited to dream. If the sensory stimulus is not always externally induced, it may be instead a stimulus proceeding from the internal organs, a so-called somatic stimulus. This conjecture is obvious, and it corresponds to the most popular conception of the origin of dreams. Dreams come from the stomach, one often hears it said. Unfortunately it may be assumed here again that the cases are frequent in which the somatic stimulus which operated during the night can no longer be traced after waking, and has thus become unverifiable. But let us not overlook the fact that many recognized experiences testify to the derivation of dreams from the somatic stimulus. It is in general indubitable that the condition of the internal organs can influence the dream. The relation of many a dream content to a distention of the bladder or to an excited condition of the genital organs, is so clear that it cannot be mistaken. From these transparent cases one can proceed to others in which, from the content of the dream, at least a justifiable conjecture may be made that such somatic stimuli have been operative, inasmuch as there is something in this content which may be conceived as elaboration, representation, interpretation of the stimuli. The dream investigator Schirmer (1861) insisted with particular emphasis on the derivation of the dream from organic stimuli, and cited several splendid examples in proof. For example, in a dream he sees "two rows of beautiful boys with blonde hair and delicate complexions stand opposite each other in preparation for a fight, fall upon each other, seize each other, take up the old position again, and repeat the whole performance;" here the interpretation of these rows of boys as teeth is plausible in itself, and it seems to become convincing when after this scene the dreamer "pulls a long tooth out of his jaws." The interpretation of "long, narrow, winding corridors" as intestinal stimuli, seems sound and confirms Schirmer's assertion that the dream above all seeks to represent the stimulus-producing organ by means of objects resembling it.

Thus we must be prepared to admit that the internal stimuli may play the same role in the dream as the external. Unfortunately, their evaluation is subject to the same difficulties as those we have already encountered. In a large number of cases the interpretation of the stimuli as somatic remains uncertain and undemonstrable. Not all dreams, but only a certain portion of them, arouse the suspicion that an internal organic stimulus was concerned in their causation. And finally, the internal stimuli will be as little able as the external sensory stimuli to explain any more of the dream than pertains to the direct reaction to the stimuli. The origin, therefore, of the rest of the dream remains obscure.

Let us, however, notice a peculiarity of dream life which becomes apparent in the study of these effects of stimuli. The dream does not simply reproduce the stimulus, but it elaborates it, it plays upon it, places it in a sequence of relationships, replaces it with something else. That is a side of dream activity which must interest us because it may lead us closer to the nature of the dream. If one does something under stimulation, then this stimulation need not exhaust the act. Shakespeare's *Macbeth*, for example, is a drama created on the occasion of the coronation of the King who for the first time wore upon his head the crown symbolizing the union of three countries. But does this historical occasion cover the content of the drama, does it explain its greatness and its riddle? Perhaps the external and internal stimuli, acting upon the sleeper, are only the incitors of the dream, of whose nature nothing is betrayed to us from our knowledge of that fact.

The other element common to dreams, their psychic peculiarity, is on the one hand hard to comprehend, and on the other hand offers no point for further investigation. In dreams we perceive a thing for the most part in visual forms. Can the stimuli furnish a solution for this fact? Is it actually the stimulus which we experience? Why, then, is the experience visual when optic stimulation incited the dream only in the rarest cases? Or can it be proved, when we dream speeches, that during sleep a conversation or sounds resembling it reached our ear? This possibility I venture decisively to reject.

If, from the common elements of dreams, we get no further, then let us see what we can do with their differences. Dreams are often senseless, blurred, absurd; but there are some that are meaningful, sober, sensible. Let us see if the latter, the sensible dreams, can give some information concerning the senseless ones. I will give you the most recent sensible dream which was told me, the dream of a young man: "I was promenading in Kärtner Street, met Mr. X. there, whom I accompanied for a bit, and then I went to a restaurant. Two ladies and a gentleman seated themselves at my table. I was annoyed at this at first, and would not look at them. Then I did look, and found that they were quite pretty." The dreamer adds that the evening before the dream he had really been in Kärtner Street, which is his usual route, and that he had met Mr. X. there. The other portion of the dream is no direct reminiscence, but bears a certain resemblance to a previous experience. Or another meaningful dream, that of a lady. "Her husband asks, 'Doesn't the piano need tuning?' She: 'It is not worth while; it has to be newly lined.'" This dream reproduces without much alteration a conversation which took place the day before between herself and her husband. What can we learn from these two sober dreams? Nothing but that you find them to be reproductions of daily life or ideas connected therewith. This would at least be something if it could be stated of all dreams. There is no question, however, that this applies to only a minority of dreams. In most dreams there is no sign of any connection with the previous day, and no light is thereby cast on the senseless and absurd dream. We know only that we have struck a new problem. We wish to know not only what it is that the dream says, but when, as in our examples, the dream speaks plainly, we also wish to know why and wherefore this recent experience is repeated in the dream.

I believe you are as tired as I am of continuing attempts like these. We see, after all, that the greatest interest in a problem is inadequate if one does not know a path which will lead to a solution. Up to this point we have not found this path. Experimental psychology gave us nothing but a few very valuable pieces of information concerning the meaning of stimuli as dream incitors. We need expect nothing from philosophy except that lately it has taken haughtily to pointing out to us the intellectual inferiority of our object. Let us not apply to the occult sciences for help. History and popular tradition tell us that the dream is meaningful and significant; it sees into the future. Yet that is hard to accept and surely not demonstrable. Thus our first efforts end in entire helplessness.

Unexpectedly we get a hint from a quarter toward which we have not yet looked. Colloquial usage—which after all is not an accidental thing but the remnant of ancient knowledge, though it should not be made use of without caution—our speech, that is to say, recognizes something which curiously enough it calls "day dreaming." Day dreams are phantasies. They are very common phenomena, again observable in the normal as well as in the sick, and access to their study is open to everyone in his own person. The most conspicuous feature about these phantastic productions is that they have received the name "day dreams," for they share neither of the two common elements of dreams. Their name contradicts the relation to the sleeping condition, and as regards the second common element, one does not experience or hallucinate anything, one only imagines it. One knows that it is a phantasy, that one is not seeing but thinking the thing. These day dreams appear in the period before puberty, often as early as the last years of childhood, continue into the years of maturity, are then either given up or retained through life. The content of these phantasies is dominated by very transparent motives. They are scenes and events in which the egoistic, ambitious and power-seeking desires of the individual find satisfaction. With young men the ambition phantasies generally prevail; in women, the erotic, since they have banked their ambition on success in love. But often enough the erotic desire appears in the background with men too; all the heroic deeds and incidents are after all meant only to win the admiration and favor of women. Otherwise these day dreams are very manifold and undergo changing fates. They are either, each in turn, abandoned after a short time and replaced by a new one, or they are retained, spun out into long stories, and adapted to changes in daily circumstances. They move with the time, so to speak, and receive from it a "time mark" which testifies to the influence of the new situation. They are the raw material of poetic production, for out of his day dreams the poet, with certain transformations, disguises and omissions, makes the situations which he puts into his novels, romances and dramas. The hero of the day dreams, however, is always the individual himself, either directly or by means of a transparent identification with another.

Perhaps day dreams bear this name because of the similarity of their relation to reality, in order to indicate that their content is as little to be taken for real as that of dreams. Perhaps, however, this identity of names does nevertheless rest on a characteristic of the dream which is still unknown to us, perhaps even one of those characteristics which we are seeking. It is possible, on the other hand, that we are wrong in trying to read a meaning into this similarity of designation. Yet that can only be cleared up later.

SIXTH LECTURE

THE DREAM

Hypothesis and Technique of Interpretation

WE must find a new path, a new method, in order to proceed with the investigation of the dream. I shall now make an obvious suggestion. Let us assume as a hypothesis for everything which follows, that *the dream is not a somatic but a psychic phenomenon*. You appreciate the significance of that statement, but what justification have we for making it? None; but that alone need not deter us from making it. The matter stands thus: If the dream is a somatic phenomenon, it does not concern us. It can be of interest to us only on the supposition that it is a *psychic* phenomenon. Let us therefore work upon that assumption in order to see what comes of it. The result of our labor will determine whether we are to hold to this assumption and whether we may, in fact, consider it in turn a result. What is it that we really wish to achieve, to what end are we working? It is what one usually seeks to attain in the sciences, an understanding of phenomena, the creation of relationships between them, and ultimately, if possible, the extension of our control over them.

Let us then proceed with the work on the assumption that the dream is a psychic phenomenon. This makes it an achievement and expression of the dreamer, but one that tells us nothing, one that we do not understand. What do you do when I make a statement you do not understand? You ask for an explanation, do you not? Why may we not do the same thing here, *ask the dreamer to give us the meaning of his dream*?

If you will remember, we were in this same situation once before. It was when we were investigating errors, a case of a slip of the tongue. Someone said: "*Da sind dinge zum vorschwein gekommen*," whereupon we asked—no, luckily, not we, but others, persons in no way associated with psychoanalysis—these persons asked him what he meant by this unintelligible talk. He immediately answered that he had intended to say "*Das waren schweinereien*," but that he had suppressed this intention, in favor of the other, more gentle "*Da sind dinge zum vorschein gekommen*."[23] I explained to you at the time that this inquiry was typical of every psychoanalytical investigation, and now you understand that psychoanalysis follows the technique, as far as possible, of having the subjects themselves discover the solutions of their riddles. The dreamer himself, then, is to tell us the meaning of his dream.

It is common knowledge, however, that this is not such an easy matter with dreams. In the case of slips, our method worked in a number of cases, but we encountered some where the subject did not wish to say anything—in fact, indignantly rejected the answer that we suggested. Instances of the first method are entirely lacking in the case of dreams; the dreamer always says he knows nothing. He cannot deny our interpretation, for we have none. Shall we then give up the attempt? Since he knows nothing and we know nothing and a third person surely knows nothing, it looks as though there were no possibility of discovering anything. If you wish, discontinue the investigation. But if you are of another mind, you can accompany me on the way. For I assure you, it is very possible, in fact, probable, that the dreamer does know what his dream means, but does *not know that he knows, and therefore believes he does not know.*

You will point out to me that I am again making an assumption, the second in this short discourse, and that I am greatly reducing the credibility of my claim. On the assumption that the dream is a psychic phenomenon, on the further assumption that there are unconscious things in man which he knows without knowing that he knows, etc.—we need only realize clearly the intrinsic improbability of each of these two assumptions, and we shall calmly turn our attention from the conclusions to be derived from such premises.

Yet, ladies and gentlemen, I have not invited you here to delude you or to conceal anything from you. I did, indeed, announce a *General Introduction to Psychoanalysis*, but I did not intend the title to convey that I was an oracle, who would show you a finished product with all the difficulties carefully concealed, all the gaps filled in and all the doubts glossed over, so that you might peacefully believe you had learned something new. No, precisely because you are beginners, I wanted to show you our science as it is, with all its hills and pitfalls, demands and considerations. For I know that it is the same in all sciences, and must be so in their beginnings particularly. I know, too, that teaching as a rule endeavors to hide these difficulties and these incompletely developed phases from the student. But that will not do in psychoanalysis. I have, as a matter of fact, made two assumptions, one within the other, and he who finds the whole too troublesome and too uncertain or is accustomed to greater security or more elegant derivations, need go no further with us. What I mean is, he should leave psychological problems entirely alone, for it must be apprehended that he will not find the sure and safe way he is prepared to go, traversable. Then, too, it is superfluous for a science that has something to offer to plead for auditors and adherents. Its results must create its atmosphere, and it must then bide its time until these have attracted attention to themselves.

I would warn those of you, however, who care to continue, that my two assumptions are not of equal worth. The first, that the dream is a psychic phenomenon, is the assumption we wish to prove by the results of our work. The other has already been proved in another field, and I take the liberty only of transferring it from that field to our problem.

Where, in what field of observation shall we seek the proof that there is in man a knowledge of which he is not conscious, as we here wish to assume in the case of the dreamer? That would be a remarkable, a surprising fact, one which would change our understanding of the psychic life, and which would have no need to hide itself. To name it would be to destroy it, and yet it pretends to be something real, a contradiction in terms. Nor does it hide itself. It is no result of the fact itself that we are ignorant of its existence and have not troubled sufficiently about it. That is just as little our fault as the fact that all these psychological problems are condemned by persons who have kept away from all observations and experiments which are decisive in this respect.

The proof appeared in the field of hypnotic phenomena. When, in the year 1889, I was a witness to the extraordinarily enlightening demonstrations of Siebault and Bernheim in Nancy, I witnessed also the following experiment: If one placed a man in the somnambulistic state, allowed him to have all manner of hallucinatory experience, and then woke him up, it appeared in the first instance that he knew nothing about what had happened during his hypnotic sleep. Bernheim then directly invited him to relate what had happened to him during the hypnosis. He maintained he was unable to recall anything. But Bernheim insisted, he persisted, he assured him he did know, that he must recall, and, incredible though it may seem, the man wavered, began to rack his memory, recalled in a shadowy way first one of the suggested experiences, then another; the recollection became more and more complete and finally was brought forth without a gap. The fact that he had this knowledge finally, and that he had had no experiences from any other source in the meantime, permits the conclusion that he knew of these recollections in the beginning. They were merely inaccessible, he did not know that he knew them; he believed he did not know them. This is exactly what we suspect in the dreamer.

I trust you are taken by surprise by the establishment of this fact, and that you will ask me why I did not refer to this proof before in the case of the slips, where we credited the man who made a mistake in speech with intentions he knew nothing about and which he denied. "If a person believes he knows nothing concerning experiences, the memory of which, however, he retains," you might say, "it is no longer so improbable that there are also other psychic experiences within him of whose existence he is ignorant. This argument would have impressed us and advanced us in the understanding of errors." To be sure, I might then have referred to this but I reserved it for another place, where it was more necessary. Errors have in a measure explained themselves, have, in part, furnished us with the warning that we must assume the existence of psychic processes of which we know nothing, for the sake of the connection of the phenomena. In dreams we are compelled to look to other sources for explanations; and besides, I count on the fact that you will permit the inference I draw from hypnotism more readily in this instance. The condition in which we make mistakes most seem to you to be the normal one. It has no similarity to the hypnotic. On the other hand, there is a clear relationship between the hypnotic state and sleep, which is the essential condition of dreams. Hypnotism is known as artificial sleep; we say to the person whom we hypnotize, "Sleep," and the suggestions which we throw out are comparable to the dreams of natural sleep. The psychical conditions are in both cases really analogous. In natural sleep we withdraw our attention from the entire outside world; in the hypnotic, on the other hand, from the whole world with the exception of the one person who has hypnotized us, with whom we remain in touch. Furthermore, the so-called nurse's sleep in which the nurse remains in touch with the child, and can be waked only by him, is a normal counterpart of hypnotism. The transference of one of the conditions of hypnotism to natural sleep does not appear to be such a daring proceeding. The inferential assumption that there is also present in the case of the dreamer a knowledge of his dream, a knowledge which is so inaccessible that he does not believe it himself, does not seem to be made out of whole cloth. Let us note that at this point there appears a third approach to the study of the dream; from the sleep-disturbing stimuli, from the day-dreams, and now in addition, from the suggested dreams of the hypnotic state.

Now we return, perhaps with increased faith, to our problem. Apparently it is very probable that the dreamer knows of his dream; the question is, how to make it possible for him to discover this knowledge, and to impart it to us? We do not demand that he give us the meaning of his dream at once, but he will be able to discover its origin, the thought and sphere of interest from which it springs. In the case of the errors, you will remember, the man was asked how he happened to use the wrong word, "*vorschwein*," and his next idea gave us the explanation. Our dream technique is very simple, an imitation of this example. We again ask how the subject happened to have the dream, and his next statement is again to be taken as an explanation. We disregard the distinction whether the dreamer believes or does not believe he knows, and treat both cases in the same way.

This technique is very simple indeed, but I am afraid it will arouse your sharpest opposition. You will say, "a new assumption. The third! And the most improbable of all! If I ask the dreamer what he considers the explanation of his dream to be, his very next association is to be the desired explanation? But it may be he thinks of nothing at all, or his next thought may be anything at all. We cannot understand upon what we can base such anticipation. This, really, is putting too much faith in a situation where a slightly more critical attitude would be more suitable. Furthermore, a dream is not an isolated error, but consists of many elements. To which idea should we pin our faith?"

You are right in all the non-essentials. A dream must indeed be distinguished from a word slip, even in the number of its elements. The technique is compelled to consider this very carefully. Let me suggest that we separate the dream into its elements, and carry on the investigation of each element separately; then the analogy to the word-slip is again set up. You are also correct when you say that in answer to the separate dream elements no association may occur to the dreamer. There are cases in which we accept this answer, and later you will hear what those cases are. They are, oddly enough, cases in which we ourselves may have certain associations. But in general we shall contradict the dreamer when he maintains he has no associations. We shall insist that he must have some association and—we shall be justified. He will bring forth some association, any one, it makes no difference to us. He will be especially facile with certain information which might be designated as historical. He will say, "that is something that happened yesterday" (as in the two "prosaic" dreams with which we are acquainted); or, "that reminds me of something that happened recently," and in this manner we shall notice that the act of associating the dreams with recent impressions is much more frequent than we had at first supposed. Finally, the dreamer will remember occurrences more remote from the dream, and ultimately even events in the far past.

But in the essential matters you are mistaken. If you believe that we assume arbitrarily that the dreamer's next association will disclose just what we are seeking, or must lead to it, that on the contrary the association is just as likely to be entirely inconsequential, and without any connection with what we are seeking, and that it is an example of my unbounded optimism to expect anything else, then you are greatly mistaken. I have already taken the liberty of pointing out that in each one of you there is a deep-rooted belief in psychic freedom and volition, a belief which is absolutely unscientific, and which must capitulate before the claims of a determinism that controls even the psychic life. I beg of you to accept it as a fact that only this one association will occur to the person questioned. But I do not put one belief in opposition to another. It can be proved that the association, which the subject produces, is not voluntary, is not indeterminable, not unconnected with what we seek. Indeed, I discovered long ago—without, however, laying too much stress on the discovery—that even experimental psychology has brought forth this evidence.

I ask you to give your particular attention to the significance of this subject. If I invite a person to tell me what occurs to him in relation to some certain element of his dream I am asking him to abandon himself to free association, *controlled by a given premise*. This demands a special delimitation of the attention, quite different from cogitation, in fact, exclusive of cogitation. Many persons put themselves into such a state easily; others show an extraordinarily high degree of clumsiness. There is a higher level of free association again, where I omit this original premise and designate only the manner of the association, e.g., rule that the subject freely give a proper name or a number. Such an association would be more voluntary, more indeterminable, than the one called forth by our technique. But it can be shown that it is strongly determined each time by an important inner mental set which, at the moment at which it is active, is unknown to us, just as unknown as the disturbing tendencies in the case of errors and the provocative tendencies in the case of accidental occurrences.

I, and many others after me, have again and again instigated such investigations for names and numbers which occur to the subject without any restraint, and have published some results. The method is the following: Proceeding from the disclosed names, we awaken continuous associations which then are no longer entirely free, but rather are limited as are the associations to the dream elements, and this is true until the impulse is exhausted. By that time, however, the motivation and significance of the free name associations is explained. The investigations always yield the same results, the information often covers a wealth of material and necessitates lengthy elaboration. The associations to freely appearing numbers are perhaps the most significant. They follow one another so quickly and approach a hidden goal with such inconceivable certainty, that it is really startling. I want to give you an example of such a name analysis, one that, happily, involves very little material.

In the course of my treatment of a young man, I referred to this subject and mentioned the fact that despite the apparent volition it is impossible to have a name occur which does not appear to be limited by the immediate conditions, the peculiarities of the subject, and the momentary situation. He was doubtful, and I proposed that he make such an attempt immediately. I know he has especially numerous relations of every sort with women and girls, and so am of the opinion that he will have an unusually wide choice if he happens to think of a woman's name. He agrees. To my astonishment, and perhaps even more to his, no avalanche of women's names descends upon my head, but he is silent for a time, and then admits that a single name has occurred to him—and no other: *Albino.* How extraordinary, but what associations have you with this name? How many albinoes do you know? Strangely enough, he knew no albinoes, and there were no further associations with the name. One might conclude the analysis had proved a failure; but no—it was already complete; no further association was necessary. The man himself had unusually light coloring. In our talks during the cure I had frequently called him an albino in fun. We were at the time occupied in determining the feminine characteristics of his nature. He himself was the Albino, who at that moment was to him the most interesting feminine person.

In like manner, melodies, which come for no reason, show themselves conditioned by and associated with a train of thought which has a right to occupy one, yet of whose activity one is unconscious. It is easily demonstrable that the attraction to the melody is associated with the text, or its origin. But I must take the precaution not to include in this assertion really musical people, with whom, as it happens, I have had no experience. In their cases the musical meaning of the melody may have occasioned its occurrence. More often the first reason holds. I know of a young man who for a time was actually haunted by the really charming melody of the song of Paris, from *The Beautiful Helen*, until the analysis brought to his attention the fact that at that time his interest was divided between an Ida and a Helen.

If then the entirely unrestrained associations are conditioned in such a manner and are arranged in a distinct order, we are justified in concluding that associations with a single condition, that of an original premise, or starting point, may be conditioned to no less degree. The investigation does in fact show that aside from the conditioning which we have established by the premise, a second farther dependence is recognizable upon powerful affective thoughts, upon cycles of interest and complexes of whose influence we are ignorant, therefore unconscious at the time.

Associations of this character have been the subject matter of very enlightening experimental investigations, which have played a noteworthy role in the history of psychoanalysis. The Wundt school proposed the so-called association-experiment, wherein the subject is given the task of answering in the quickest possible time, with any desired reaction, to a given stimulus-word. It is then possible to study the interval of time that elapses between the stimulus and the reaction, the nature of the answer given as reaction, the possible mistake in a subsequent repetition of the same attempt, and similar matters. The Zurich School under the leadership of Bleuler and Jung, gave the explanation of the reactions following the association-experiment, by asking the subject to explain a given reaction by means of further associations, in the cases where there was anything extraordinary in the reaction. It then became apparent that these extraordinary reactions were most sharply determined by the complexes of the subject. In this matter Bleuler and Jung built the first bridge from experimental psychology to psychoanalysis.

Thus instructed, you will be able to say, "We recognize now that free associations are predetermined, not voluntary, as we had believed. We admit this also as regards the associations connected with the elements of the dream, but that is not what we are concerned with. You maintain that the associations to the dream element are determined by the unknown psychic background of this very element. We do not think that this is a proven fact. We expect, to be sure, that the association to the dream element will clearly show itself through one of the complexes of the dreamer, but what good is that to us? That does not lead us to understand the dream, but rather, as in the case of the association-experiment, to a knowledge of the so-called complexes. What have these to do with the dream?"

You are right, but you overlook one point, in fact, the very point because of which I did not choose the association-experiment as the starting point for this exposition. In this experiment the one determinate of the reaction, viz., the stimulus word, is voluntarily chosen. The reaction is then an intermediary between this stimulus word and the recently aroused complex of the subject. In the dream the stimulus word is replaced by something that itself has its origin in the psychic life of the dreamer, in sources unknown to him, hence very likely itself a product of the complex. It is not an altogether fantastic hypothesis, then, that the more remote associations, even those that are connected with the dream element, are determined by no other complex than the one which determines the dream element itself, and will lead to the disclosure of the complex.

Let me show you by another case that the situation is really as we expect it to be. Forgetting proper names is really a splendid example for the case of dream analysis; only here there is present in one person what in the dream interpretation is divided between two persons. Though I have forgotten a name temporarily I still retain the certainty that I know the name; that certainty which we could acquire for the dreamer only by way of the Bernheim experiment. The forgotten name, however, is not accessible. Cogitation, no matter how strenuous, does not help. Experience soon tells me that. But I am able each time to find one or more substitute names for the forgotten name. If such a substitute name occurs to me spontaneously then the correspondence between this situation and that of the dream analysis first becomes evident. Nor is the dream element the real thing, but only a substitute for something else, for what particular thing I do not know, but am to discover by means of the dream analysis. The difference lies only in this, that in forgetting a name I recognize the substitute automatically as unsuitable, while in the dream element we must acquire this interpretation with great labor. When a name is forgotten, too, there is a way to go from the substitute to the unknown reality, to arrive at the forgotten name. If I centre my attention on the substitute name and allow further associations to accumulate, I arrive in a more or less roundabout way at the forgotten name, and discover that the spontaneous substitute names, together with those called up by me, have a certain connection with the forgotten name, were conditioned by it.

I want to show you an analysis of this type. One day I noticed that I could not recall the name of the little country in the Riviera of which Monte Carlo is the capital. It is very annoying, but it is true. I steep myself in all my knowledge about this country, think of Prince Albert, of the house of Lusignan, of his marriages, his preference for deep-sea study, and anything else I can think of, but to no avail. So I give up the thinking, and in place of the lost name allow substitute names to suggest themselves. They come quickly—Monte Carlo itself, then Piedmont, Albania, Montevideo, Colico. Albania is the first to attract my attention, it is replaced by Montenegro, probably because of the contrast between black and white. Then I see that four of these substitutes contain the same syllable *mon*. I suddenly have the forgotten word, and cry aloud, "*Monaco*." The substitutes really originated in the forgotten word, the four first from the first syllable, the last brings back the sequence of syllables and the entire final syllable. In addition, I am also able easily to discover what it was that took the name from my memory for a time. Monaco is also the Italian name of Munich; this latter town exerted the inhibiting influence.

The example is pretty enough, but too simple. In other cases we must add to the first substitute names a long line of associations, and then the analogy to the dream interpretation becomes clearer. I have also had such experiences. Once when a stranger invited me to drink Italian wine with him, it so happened in the hostelry that he forgot the name of the wine he had intended to order just because he had retained a most pleasant memory of it. Out of a profusion of dissimilar substitute associations which came to him in the place of the forgotten name, I was able to conclude that the memory of some one named Hedwig had deprived him of the name of the wine, and he actually confirmed not only that he had first tasted this wine in the company of a Hedwig, but he also, as a result of this declaration, recollected the name again. He was at the time happily married, and this Hedwig belonged to former times, not now recalled with pleasure.

What is possible in forgetting names must work also in dream interpretation, viz., making the withheld actuality accessible by means of substitutions and through connecting associations. As exemplified by name-forgetting, we may conclude that in the case of the associations to the dream element they will be determined as well by the dream element as by its unknown essential. Accordingly, we have advanced a few steps in the formulation of our dream technique.

SEVENTH LECTURE

THE DREAM

W E have not studied the problem of errors in vain. Thanks to our efforts in this field, under the conditions known to you, we have evolved two different things, a conception of the elements of the dream and a technique for dream interpretation. The conception of the dream element goes to show something unreal, a substitute for something else, unknown to the dreamer, similar to the tendency of errors, a substitute for something the dreamer knows but cannot approach. We hope to transfer the same conception to the whole dream, which consists of just such elements. Our method consists of calling up, by means of free associations, other substitute formations in addition to these elements, from which we divine what is hidden.

Let me ask you to permit a slight change in our nomenclature which will greatly increase the flexibility of our vocabulary. Instead of hidden, unapproachable, unreal, let us give a truer description and say inaccessible or unknown to the consciousness of the dreamer. By this we mean only what the connection with the lost word or with the interfering intention of the error can suggest to you, namely, unconscious *for the time being*. Naturally in contrast to this we may term *conscious* the elements of the dream itself and the substitute formations just gained by association. As yet there is absolutely no theoretical construction implied in this nomenclature. The use of the word unconscious as a suitable and intelligible descriptive epithet is above criticism.

If we transfer our conception from a single element to the entire dream, we find that the dream as a whole is a distorted substitute for something else, something unconscious. To discover this unconscious thing is the task of dream interpretation. From this, three important rules, which we must observe in the work of dream interpretation, are straightway derived:

1. What the dream seems to say, whether it be sensible or absurd, clear or confused is not our concern, since it can under no condition be that unconscious content we are seeking. Later we shall have to observe an obvious limitation of this rule. 2. The awakening of substitute formations for each element shall be the sole object of our work. We shall not reflect on these, test their suitability or trouble how far they lead away from the element of the dream. 3. We shall wait until the hidden unconscious we are seeking appears of itself, as the missing word *Monaco* in the experiment which we have described.

Now we can understand, too, how unimportant it is how much, how little, above all, how accurately or how indifferently the dream is remembered. For the dream which is remembered is not the real one, but a distorted substitute, which is to help us approach the real dream by awakening other substitute formations and by making the unconscious in the dream conscious. Therefore if our recollection of the dream was faulty, it has simply brought about a further distortion of this substitute, a distortion which cannot, however, be unmotivated.

One can interpret one's own dreams as well as those of others. One learns even more from these, for the process yields more proof. If we try this, we observe that something impedes the work. Haphazard ideas arise, but we do not let them have their way. Tendencies to test and to choose make themselves felt. As an idea occurs, we say to ourselves "No, that does not fit, that does not belong here"; of a second "that is too senseless"; of a third, "this is entirely beside the point"; and one can easily observe how the ideas are stifled and suppressed by these objections, even before they have become entirely clear. On the one hand, therefore, too much importance is attached to the dream elements themselves; on the other, the result of free association is vitiated by the process of selection. If you are not interpreting the dream alone, if you allow someone else to interpret it for you, you will soon discover another motive which induces you to make this forbidden choice. At times you say to yourself, "No, this idea is too unpleasant, I either will not or cannot divulge this."

Clearly these objections are a menace to the success of our work. We must guard against them, in our own case by the firm resolve not to give way to them; and in the interpretation of the dreams of others by making the hard and fast rule for them, never to omit any idea from their account, even if one of the following four objections should arise: that is, if it should seem too unimportant, absurd, too irrelevant or too embarrassing to relate. The dreamer promises to obey this rule, but it is annoying to see how poorly he keeps his promise at times. At first we account for this by supposing that in spite of the authoritative assurance which has been given to the dreamer, he is not impressed with the importance of free association, and plan perhaps to win his theoretic approval by giving him papers to read or by sending him to lectures which are to make him a disciple of our views concerning free association. But we are deterred from such blunders by the observation that, in one's own case, where convictions may certainly be trusted, the same critical objections arise against certain ideas, and can only be suppressed subsequently, upon second thought, as it were.

Instead of becoming vexed at the disobedience of the dreamer, these experiences can be turned to account in teaching something new, something which is the more important the less we are prepared for it. We understand that the task of interpreting dreams is carried on against a certain *resistance* which manifests itself by these critical objections. This resistance is independent of the theoretical conviction of the dreamer. Even more is apparent. We discover that such a critical objection is never justified. On the contrary, those ideas which we are so anxious to suppress, prove *without exception* to be the most important, the most decisive, in the search for the unconscious. It is even a mark of distinction if an idea is accompanied by such an objection.

This resistance is something entirely new, a phenomenon which we have found as a result of our hypotheses although it was not originally included in them. We are not too pleasantly surprised by this new factor in our problem. We suspect that it will not make our work any easier. It might even tempt us to abandon our entire work in connection with the dream. Such an unimportant thing as the dream and in addition such difficulties instead of a smooth technique! But from another point of view, these same difficulties may prove fascinating, and suggest that the work is worth the trouble. Whenever we try to penetrate to the hidden unconscious, starting out from the substitute which the dream element represents, we meet with resistance. Hence, we are justified in supposing that something of weight must be hidden behind the substitute. What other reason could there be for the difficulties which are maintained for purposes of concealment? If a child does not want to open his clenched fist, he is certainly hiding something he ought not to have.

Just as soon as we bring the dynamic representation of resistance into our consideration of the case, we must realize that this factor is something quantitatively variable. There may be greater or lesser resistances and we are prepared to see these differences in the course of our work. We may perhaps connect this with another experience found in the work of dream interpretation. For sometimes only one or two ideas serve to carry us from the dream element to its unconscious aspect, while at other times long chains of associations and the suppression of many critical objections are necessary. We shall note that these variations are connected with the variable force of resistance. This observation is probably correct. If resistance is slight, then the substitute is not far removed from the unconscious, but strong resistance carries with it a great distortion of the unconscious and in addition a long journey back to it.

Perhaps the time has come to take a dream and try out our method to see if our faith in it shall be confirmed. But which dream shall we choose? You cannot imagine how hard it is for me to decide, and at this point I cannot explain the source of the difficulty. Of course, there must be dreams which, as a whole, have suffered slight distortion, and it would be best to start with one of these. But which dreams are the least distorted? Those which are sensible and not confused, of which I have already given you two examples? This would be a gross misunderstanding. Testing shows that these dreams have suffered by distortion to an exceptionally high degree. But if I take the first best dream, regardless of certain necessary conditions, you would probably be very much disappointed. Perhaps we should have to note such an abundance of ideas in connection with single elements of dream that it would be absolutely impossible to review the work in perspective. If we write the dream out and confront it with the written account of all the ideas which arise in connection with it, these may easily amount to a reiteration of the text of the dream. It would therefore seem most practical to choose for analysis several short dreams of which each one can at least reveal or confirm something. This is what we shall decide upon, provided experience should not point out where we shall really find slightly distorted dreams.

But I know of another way to simplify matters, one which, moreover, lies in our path. Instead of attempting the interpretation of entire dreams, we shall limit ourselves to single dream elements and by observing a series of examples we shall see how these are explained by the application of our method.

1. A lady relates that as a child she often dreamt "*that God had a pointed paper hat on his head.*" How do you expect to understand that without the help of the dreamer? Why, it sounds quite absurd. It is no longer absurd when the lady testifies that as a child she was frequently made to wear such a hat at the table, because she could not help stealing glances at the plates of her brothers and sisters to see if one of them had gotten more than she. The hat was therefore supposed to act as a sort of blinder. This explanation was moreover historic, and given without the least difficulty. The meaning of this fragment and of the whole brief dream, is clear with the help of a further idea of the dreamer. "Since I had heard that God was all-knowing and all-seeing," she said, "the dream can only mean that I know everything and see everything just as God does, even when they try to prevent me." This example is perhaps too simple.

2. A sceptical patient has a longer dream, in which certain people happen to tell her about my book concerning laughter and praise it highly. Then something is mentioned about a certain "*'canal,' perhaps another book in which 'canal' occurs, or something else with the word 'canal' ... she doesn't know ... it is all confused.*"

Now you will be inclined to think that the element "canal" will evade interpretation because it is so vague. You are right as to the supposed difficulty, but it is not difficult because it is vague, but rather it is vague for a different reason, the same reason which also makes the interpretation difficult. The dreamer can think of nothing concerning the word canal, I naturally can think of nothing. A little while later, as a matter of fact on the next day, she tells me that something occurred to her that *may perhaps* be related to it, a joke that she has heard. On a ship between Dover and Calais a well-known author is conversing with an Englishman, who quoted the following proverb in a certain connection: "*Du sublime au ridicule, il n'y a qu'un pas.*"[24] The author answers, "*Oui, le pas de Calais,*"[25] with which he wishes to say that he finds France sublime and England ridiculous. But the "*Pas de Calais*" is really a canal, namely, the English Channel. Do I think that this idea has anything to do with the dream? Certainly, I believe that it really gives the solution to the puzzling dream fragments. Or can you doubt that this joke was already present in the dream, as the unconscious factor of the element, "canal." Can you take it for granted that it was subsequently added to it? The idea testifies to the scepticism which is concealed behind her obtrusive admiration, and the resistance is probably the common reason for both phenomena, for the fact that the idea came so hesitatingly and that the decisive element of the dream turned out to be so vague. Kindly observe at this point the relation of the dream element to its unconscious factor. It is like a small part of the unconscious, like an allusion to it; through its isolation it became quite unintelligible.

3. A patient dreams, in the course of a longer dream: "*Around a table of peculiar shape several members of his family are sitting, etc.*" In connection with this table, it occurs to him that he saw such a piece of furniture during a visit to a certain family. Then his thoughts continue: In this family a peculiar relation had existed between father and son, and soon he adds to this that as a matter of fact the same

relation exists between himself and his father. The table is therefore taken up into the dream to designate this parallel.

This dreamer had for a long time been familiar with the claims of dream interpretation. Otherwise he might have taken exception to the fact that so trivial a detail as the shape of a table should be taken as the basis of the investigation. As a matter of fact we judge nothing in the dream as accidental or indifferent, and we expect to reach our conclusion by the explanation of just such trivial and unmotivated details. Perhaps you will be surprised that the dream work should arouse the thought "we are in exactly the same position as they are," just by the choice of the table. But even this becomes clear when you learn that the name of the family in question is *Tischler*. By permitting his own family to sit at such a table, he intends to express that they too are *Tischler*. Please note how, in relating such a dream interpretation, one must of necessity become indiscreet. Here you have arrived at one of the difficulties in the choice of examples that I indicated before. I could easily have substituted another example for this one, but would probably have avoided this indiscretion at the cost of committing another one in its place.

The time has come to introduce two new terms, which we could have used long ago. We shall call that which the dream relates, the manifest content of the dream; that which is hidden, which we can only reach by the analysis of ideas we shall call latent dream thoughts. We may now consider the connection between the manifest dream content and the latent dream thoughts as they are revealed in these examples. Many different connections can exist. In examples 1 and 2 the manifest content is also a constituent part of the latent thought, but only a very small part of it. A small piece of a great composite psychic structure in the unconscious dream thought has penetrated into the manifest dream, like a fragment of it, or in other cases, like an allusion to it, like a catchword or an abbreviation in the telegraphic code. The interpretation must mould this fragment, or indication, into a whole, as was done most successfully in example 2. One sort of distortion of which the dream mechanism consists is therefore substitution by means of a fragment or an allusion. In the third, moreover, we must recognize another relation which we shall see more clearly and distinctly expressed in the following examples:

4. The dreamer "*pulls a certain woman of his acquaintance from behind a bed.*" He finds the meaning of this dream element himself by his first association. It means: This woman "has a pull" with him.[26]

5. Another man dreams that "*his brother is in a closet.*" The first association substitutes *clothes-press* for closet, and the second gives the meaning: his brother is *close-pressed* for money.[27]

6. The dreamer "*climbs a mountain from the top of which he has an extraordinarily distant view.*" This sounds quite sensible; perhaps there is nothing about it that needs interpretation, and it is simply necessary to find out which reminiscence this dream touches upon and why it was recalled. But you are mistaken; it is evident that this dream requires interpretation as well as any other which is confused. For no previous mountain climbing of his own occurs to the

dreamer, but he remembers that an acquaintance of his is publishing a "*Rundschau*," which deals with our relation to the furthermost parts of the earth. The latent dream thought is therefore in this case an identification of the dreamer with the "*Rundschauer*."

Here you find a new type of connection between the manifest content and the latent dream element. The former is not so much a distortion of the latter as a representation of it, a plastic concrete perversion that is based on the sound of the word. However, it is for this very reason again a distortion, for we have long ago forgotten from which concrete picture the word has arisen, and therefore do not recognize it by the image which is substituted for it. If you consider that the manifest dream consists most often of visual images, and less frequently of thoughts and words, you can imagine that a very particular significance in dream formation is attached to this sort of relation. You can also see that in this manner it becomes possible to create substitute formations for a great number of abstract thoughts in the manifest dream, substitutions that serve the purpose of further concealment all the same. This is the technique of our picture puzzle. What the origin is of the semblance of wit which accompanies such representations is a particular question which we need not touch upon at this time.

A fourth type of relation between the manifest and the latent dream cannot be dealt with until its cue in the technique has been given. Even then I shall not have given you a complete enumeration, but it will be sufficient for our purpose.

Have you the courage to venture upon the interpretation of an entire dream? Let us see if we are well enough equipped for this undertaking. Of course, I shall not choose one of the most obscure, but one nevertheless that shows in clear outline the general characteristics of a dream.

A young woman who has been married for many years dreams: "*She is sitting in the theatre with her husband; one side of the orchestra is entirely unoccupied. Her husband tells her that Elise L. and her bridegroom had also wished to come, but had only been able to procure poor seats, three for 1 Fl., 50 Kr. and those of course they could not take. She thinks this is no misfortune for them.*"

The first thing that the dreamer has to testify is that the occasion for the dream is touched upon in its manifest content. Her husband had really told her that Elise L., an acquaintance of about her age, had become engaged. The dream is the reaction to this news. We already know that in the case of many dreams it is easy to trace such a cause to the preceding day, and that the dreamer often gives these deductions without any difficulty. The dreamer also places at our disposal further information for other parts of the manifest dream content. Whence the detail that one side of the orchestra is unoccupied? It is an allusion to an actual occurrence of the previous week. She had made up her mind to go to a certain performance and had procured tickets in advance, so much in advance that she had been forced to pay a preference tax.[28] When she arrived at the theatre, she saw how needless had been her anxiety, for *one side of the orchestra was almost empty*. She could have bought the tickets on the day of the performance itself. Her husband would not stop teasing her about her excessive haste. Whence the 1 Fl. 50 Kr.? From a very different connection that has nothing to do with the former, but which also alludes to an occurrence of the previous day. Her sister-in-law had received 150 florins as a present from her husband, and knew no better, the poor goose, than to hasten to the jeweler and spend the money on a piece of jewelry. Whence the number 3? She can think of nothing in connection with this unless one stresses the association that the bride, Elise L., is only three months younger than she herself, who has been married for almost ten years. And the absurdity of buying three tickets for two people? She says nothing of this, and indeed denies all further associations or information.

But she has given us so much material in her few associations, that it becomes possible to derive the latent dream thought from it. It must strike us that in her remarks concerning the dream, time elements which constitute a common element in the various parts of this material appear at several points. She attended to the tickets *too soon*, took them *too hastily*, so that she had to pay more than usual for them; her sister-in-law likewise *hastened* to carry her money to the jeweler's to buy a piece of jewelry, just as if she might *miss* it. Let us add to the expressions "*too early*," "*precipitately*," which are emphasized so strongly, the occasion for the dream, namely, that her friend only three months younger than herself had even now gotten a good husband, and the criticism expressed in the condemnation of her sister-in-law, that it was *foolish* to hurry so. Then the following construction of the latent dream thought, for which the manifest dream is a badly distorted substitute, comes to us almost spontaneously:

"How *foolish* it was of me to hurry so in marrying! Elise's example shows me that I could have gotten a husband later too." (The precipitateness is represented by her own behavior in buying the tickets, and that of her sister-in-law in purchasing jewelry. Going to the theatre was substituted for getting married. This appears to have been the main thought; and perhaps we may continue, though with less certainty, because the analysis in these parts is not supported by statements of the dreamer.) "And I would have gotten 100 times as much for my money." (150 Fl. is 100 times as much as 1 Fl. 50 Kr.). If we might substitute the dowry for the money, then it would mean that one buys a husband with a dowry; the jewelry as well as the poor seats would represent the husband. It would be even more desirable if the fragment "3 seats" had something to do with a husband. But our understanding does not penetrate so far. We have only guessed that the dream expresses her *disparagement* of her own husband, and her regret at having *married so early*.

It is my opinion that we are more surprised and confused than satisfied by the result of this first dream interpretation. We are swamped by more impressions than we can master. We see that the teachings of dream interpretation are not easily exhausted. Let us hasten to select those points that we recognize as giving us new, sound insight.

In the first place, it is remarkable that in the latent thought the main emphasis falls on the element of haste; in the manifest dream there is absolutely no mention of this to be found. Without the analysis we should not have had any idea that this element was of any importance at all. So it seems possible that just the main thing, the central point of the unconscious thoughts, may be absent in the manifest dream. Because of this, the original impression in the dream must of necessity be entirely changed. Secondly: In the dream there is a senseless combination, 3 for 1 Fl. 50 Kr.; in the dream thought we divine the sentence, "It was senseless (to marry so early)." Can one deny that this thought, "It was senseless," was represented in the manifest dream by the introduction of an absurd element? Thirdly: Comparison will show that the relation between the manifest and latent elements is not simple, certainly not of such a sort that a manifest element is always substituted for the latent. There must rather be a quantitative relationship between the two groups, according to which a manifest element may represent several latent ones, or a latent element represented by several manifest elements.

Much that is surprising might also be said of the sense of the dream and the dreamer's reaction to it. She acknowledges the interpretation but wonders at it. She did not know that she disparaged her husband so, and she did not know why she should disparage him to such a degree. There is still much that is incomprehensible. I really believe that we are not yet fully equipped for dream interpretation, and that we must first receive further instruction and preparation.

EIGHTH LECTURE

THE DREAM

Dreams of Childhood

W E think we have advanced too rapidly. Let us go back a little. Before our last attempt to overcome the difficulties of dream distortion through our technique, we had decided that it would be best to avoid them by limiting ourselves only to those dreams in which distortion is either entirely absent or of trifling importance, if there are such. But here again we digress from the history of the evolution of our knowledge, for as a matter of fact we become aware of dreams entirely free of distortion only after the consistent application of our method of interpretation and after complete analysis of the distorted dream.

The dreams we are looking for are found in children. They are short, clear, coherent, easy to understand, unambiguous, and yet unquestionable dreams. But do not think that all children's dreams are like this. Dream distortion makes its appearance very early in childhood, and dreams of children from five to eight years of age have been recorded that showed all the characteristics of later dreams. But if you will limit yourselves to the age beginning with conscious psychic activity, up to the fourth or fifth year, you will discover a series of dreams that are of a so-called infantile character. In a later period of childhood you will be able to find some dreams of this nature occasionally. Even among adults, dreams that closely resemble the typically infantile ones occur under certain conditions.

From these children's dreams we gain information concerning the nature of dreams with great ease and certainty, and we hope it will prove decisive and of universal application.

1. For the understanding of these dreams we need no analysis, no technical methods. We need not question the child that is giving an account of his dream. But one must add to this a story taken from the life of the child. An experience of the previous day will always explain the dream to us. The dream is a sleep-reaction of psychic life upon these experiences of the day.

We shall now consider a few examples so that we may base our further deductions upon them.

a). A boy of 22 months is to present a basket of cherries as a birthday gift. He plainly does so very unwillingly, although they promise him that he will get some of them himself. The next morning he relates as his dream, "*Hermann eat all cherries.*"

b). A little girl of three and a quarter years makes her first trip across a lake. At the landing she does not want to leave the boat and cries bitterly. The time of the trip seems to her to have passed entirely too rapidly. The next morning she says, "*Last night I rode on the lake.*" We may add the supplementary fact that this trip lasted longer.

c). A boy of five and a quarter years is taken on an excursion into the Escherntal near Hallstatt. He had heard that Hallstatt lay at the foot of the Dachstein, and had shown great interest in this mountain. From his home in Aussee there was a beautiful view of the Dachstein, and with a telescope one could discern the Simonyhütte upon it. The child had tried again and again to see it through the telescope, with what result no one knew. He started on the excursion in a joyously expectant mood. Whenever a new mountain came in sight the boy asked, "Is that the Dachstein?" The oftener this question was answered in the negative, the more moody he became; later he became entirely silent and would not take part in a small climb to a waterfall. They thought he was overtired, but the next morning, he said quite happily, "*Last night I dreamed that we were in the Simonyhütte.*" It was with this expectation, therefore, that he had taken part in the excursion. The only detail he gave was one he had heard before, "you had to climb steps for six hours."

These three dreams will suffice for all the information we desire.

2. We see that children's dreams are not meaningless; they are *intelligible, significant, psychic acts*. You will recall what I represented to you as the medical opinion concerning the dream, the simile of untrained fingers wandering aimlessly over the keys of the piano. You cannot fail to see how decidedly these dreams of childhood are opposed to this conception. But it would be strange indeed if the child brought forth complete psychic products in sleep, while the adult in the same

condition contents himself with spasmodic reactions. Indeed, we have every reason to attribute the more normal and deeper sleep to the child.

3. Dream distortion is lacking in these dreams, therefore they need no interpretation. The manifest and latent dreams are merged. *Dream distortion is therefore not inherent in the dream.* I may assume that this relieves you of a great burden. But upon closer consideration we shall have to admit of a tiny bit of distortion, a certain differentiation between manifest dream content and latent dream thought, even in these dreams.

4. The child's dream is a reaction to an experience of the day, which has left behind it a regret, a longing or an unfulfilled desire. *The dream brings about the direct unconcealed fulfillment of this wish.* Now recall our discussions concerning the importance of the role of external or internal bodily stimuli as disturbers of sleep, or as dream producers. We learned definite facts about this, but could only explain a very small number of dreams in this way. In these children's dreams nothing points to the influence of such somatic stimuli; we cannot be mistaken, for the dreams are entirely intelligible and easy to survey. But we need not give up the theory of physical causation entirely on this account. We can only ask why at the outset we forgot that besides the physical stimuli there are also psychic sleep-disturbing stimuli. For we know that it is these stimuli that commonly cause the disturbed sleep of adults by preventing them from producing the ideal condition of sleep, the withdrawal of interest from the world. The dreamer does not wish to interrupt his life, but would rather continue his work with the things that occupy him, and for this reason he does not sleep. The unfulfilled wish, to which he reacts by means of the dream, is the psychic sleep-disturbing stimulus for the child.

5. From this point we easily arrive at an explanation of the function of the dream. The dream, as a reaction to the psychic stimulus, must have the value of a release of this stimulus which results in its elimination and in the continuation of sleep. We do not know how this release is made possible by the dream, but we note that *the dream is not a disturber of sleep,* as calumny says, *but a guardian of sleep, whose duty it is to quell disturbances.* It is true, we think we would have slept better if we had not dreamt, but here we are wrong; as a matter of fact, we would not have slept at all without the help of the dream. That we have slept so soundly is due to the dream alone. It could not help disturbing us slightly, just as the night watchman often cannot avoid making a little noise while he drives away the rioters who would awaken us with their noise.

6. One main characteristic of the dream is that a wish is its source, and that the content of the dream is the gratification of this wish. Another equally constant feature is that the dream does not merely express a thought, but also represents the fulfillment of this wish in the form of a hallucinatory experience. "*I should like to travel on the lake,*" says the wish that excites the dream; the dream itself has as its content "*I travel on the lake.*" One distinction between the latent and manifest dream, a distortion of the latent dream thought, therefore remains even in the case of these simple children's dreams, namely, *the translation of the thought into experience.* In the interpretation of the dream it is of utmost importance that this

change be traced back. If this should prove to be an extremely common characteristic of the dream, then the above mentioned dream fragment, "*I see my brother in a closet*" could not be translated, "*My brother is close-pressed*," but rather, "I wish that my brother were close-pressed, *my brother should be close-pressed.*" Of the two universal characteristics of the dream we have cited, the second plainly has greater prospects of unconditional acknowledgment than the first. Only extensive investigation can ascertain that the cause of the dream must always be a wish, and cannot also be an anxiety, a plan or a reproach; but this does not alter the other characteristic, that the dream does not simply reproduce the stimulus but by experiencing it anew, as it were, removes, expels and settles it.

7. In connection with these characteristics of the dream we can again resume the comparison between the dream and the error. In the case of the latter we distinguish an interfering tendency and one interfered with, and the error is the compromise between the two. The dream fits into the same scheme. The tendency interfered with, in this case, can be no other than that of sleep. For the interfering tendency we substitute the psychic stimulus, the wish which strives for its fulfillment, let us say, for thus far we are not familiar with any other sleep-disturbing psychic stimulus. In this instance also the dream is the result of compromise. We sleep, and yet we experience the removal of a wish; we gratify the wish, but at the same time continue to sleep. Both are partly carried out and partly given up.

8. You will remember that we once hoped to gain access to the understanding of the dream problem by the fact that certain very transparent phantasy formations are called *day dreams*. Now these day dreams are actual wish fulfillments, fulfillments of ambitious or erotic wishes with which we are familiar; but they are conscious, and though vividly imagined, they are never hallucinatory experiences. In this instance, therefore, the less firmly established of the two main characteristics of the dream holds, while the other proves itself entirely dependent upon the condition of sleep and impossible to the waking state. In colloquial usage, therefore, there is a presentment of the fact that the fulfillment of a wish is a main characteristic of the dream. Furthermore, if the experience in the dream is a transformed representation only made possible by the condition of sleep—in other words, a sort of nocturnal day dream—then we can readily understand that the occurrence of phantasy formations can release the nocturnal stimulus and bring satisfaction. For day dreaming is an activity closely bound up in gratification and is, indeed, pursued only for this reason.

Not only this but other colloquial usages also express the same feeling. Well-known proverbs say, "The pig dreams of acorns, the goose of maize," or ask, "Of what does the hen dream? Of millet." So the proverb descends even lower than we do, from the child to the animal, and maintains that the content of a dream is the satisfaction of a need. Many turns of speech seem to point to the same thing—"dreamlike beauty," "I should never have dreamed of that," "in my wildest dreams I hadn't imagined that." This is open partisanship on the part of colloquial usage. For there are also dreams of fear and dreams of embarrassing or indifferent content, but they have not been drawn into common usage. It is true that common usage recognizes "bad" dreams, but still the dream plainly connotates to it only the beautiful wish fulfillment. There is indeed no proverb that tells us that the pig or the goose dreams of being slaughtered.

Of course it is unbelievable that the wish-fulfillment characteristic has not been noted by writers on the dream. Indeed, this was very often the case, but none of them thought of acknowledging this characteristic as universal and of making it the basis of an explanation of the dream. We can easily imagine what may have deterred them and shall discuss it subsequently.

See what an abundance of information we have gained, with almost no effort, from the consideration of children's dreams—the function of the dream as a guardian of sleep; its origin from two rival tendencies, of which the one, the longing for sleep, remains constant, while the other tries to satisfy a psychic stimulus; the proof that the dream is a significant psychic act; its two main characteristics: wish fulfillment and hallucinatory experience. And we were almost able to forget that we are engaged in psychoanalysis. Aside from its connection with errors our work has no specific connotation. Any psychologist, who is entirely ignorant of the claims of psychoanalysis, could have given this explanation of children's dreams. Why has no one done so?

If there were only infantile dreams, our problem would be solved, our task accomplished, and that without questioning the dreamer, or approaching the unconscious, and without taking free association into consideration. The continuation of our task plainly lies in this direction. We have already repeatedly had the experience that characteristics that at first seemed universally true, have subsequently held good only for a certain kind and for a certain number of dreams. It is therefore for us to decide whether the common characteristics which we have gathered from children's dreams can be applied universally, whether they also hold for those dreams that are not transparent, whose manifest content shows no connection with wishes left over from the previous day. We think that these dreams have undergone considerable distortion and for this reason are not to be judged superficially. We also suspect that for the explanation of this distortion we shall need the psychoanalytic method which we could dispense with in the understanding of children's dreams.

There is at any rate a class of dreams that are undistorted, and, just like children's dreams, are easily recognizable as wish fulfillments. It is those that are called up throughout life by the imperative needs of the body—hunger, thirst, sexual desire—hence wish fulfillments in reaction to internal physical stimuli. For this reason, I have noted the dream of a young girl, that consisted of a menu following her name (Anna F......, strawberry, huckleberry, egg-dish, pap), as a reaction to an enforced day of fasting on account of a spoiled stomach, which was directly traceable to the eating of the fruits twice mentioned in the dream. At the same time, the grandmother, whose age added to that of her grandchild would make a full seventy, had to go without food for a day on account of kidney-trouble, and dreamed the same night that she had been invited out and that the finest tid-bits had been set before her. Observations with prisoners who are allowed to go hungry, or with people who suffer privations on travels or expeditions, show that under these conditions the dreams regularly deal with the satisfaction of these needs. Otto Nordenskjold, in his book *Antarctic* (1904), testifies to the same thing concerning his crew, who were ice-bound with him during the winter (Vol. 1, page 336). "Very significant in determining the trend of our inmost thoughts were our dreams, which were never more vivid and numerous than just at this time. Even those of our comrades who ordinarily dreamed but seldom, now had long stories to tell, when in the morning we exchanged our latest experiences in that realm of phantasy. All of them dealt with that outside world that now was so far away from us, but often they fitted into our present condition. Food and drink were most often the pivots about which our dreams revolved. One of us, who excelled in going to great dinners in his sleep, was most happy whenever he could tell us in the morning that he attended a dinner of three courses; another one dreamed of tobacco, whole mountains of tobacco; still another dreamed of a ship that came along on the open sea, under full sail. One other dream deserves mention: The postman comes with the mail and gives a long explanation of why it is so late; he had delivered it to the wrong address and only after great trouble on his part had succeeded in getting it back. Of course one occupies himself with even more impossible things in sleep, but in nearly all the dreams that I myself dreamed or heard tell of, the lack of phantasy was quite striking. It would surely be of great psychological interest if all these dreams were recorded. It is easy to understand how we longed for sleep, since it could offer us everything for which each one of us felt the most burning desire." I quote further from Du Prel. "Mungo Park, who during a trip in Africa was almost exhausted, dreamed without interruption of the fertile valleys and fields of his home. Trenck, tortured by hunger in the redoubt at Magdeburg, likewise saw himself surrounded by wonderful meals, and George Back, who took part in Franklin's first expedition, dreamed regularly and consistently of luxurious meals when, as a result of terrible privations, he was nearly dead of hunger."

A man who feels great thirst at night after enjoying highly seasoned food for supper, often dreams that he is drinking. It is of course impossible to satisfy a rather strong desire for food or drink by means of the dream; from such a dream one awakes thirsty and must now drink real water. The effect of the dream is in this case practically trifling, but it is none the less clear that it was called up for the purpose of maintaining the sleep in spite of the urgent impulse to awake and to act. Dreams of satisfaction often overcome needs of a lesser intensity.

In a like manner, under the influence of sexual stimuli, the dream brings about satisfaction that shows noteworthy peculiarities. As a result of the characteristic of the sexual urge which makes it somewhat less dependent upon its object than hunger and thirst, satisfaction in a dream of pollution may be an actual one, and as a result of difficulties to be mentioned later in connection with the object, it happens especially often that the actual satisfaction is connected with confused or distorted dream content. This peculiarity of the dream of pollution, as O. Rank has observed, makes it a fruitful subject to pursue in the study of dream distortion. Moreover, all dreams of desire of adults usually contain something besides satisfaction, something that has its origin in the sources of the purely psychic stimuli, and which requires interpretation to render it intelligible.

Moreover we shall not maintain that the wish-fulfillment dreams of the infantile kind occur in adults only as reactions to the known imperative desires. We also know of short cleardreams of this sort under the influence of dominating situations that arise from unquestionably psychic sources. As, for example, in dreams of impatience, whenever a person has made preparations for a journey, for a theatrical performance, for a lecture or for a visit, and now dreams of the anticipated fulfillment of his expectations, and so arrives at his goal the night before the actual experience, in the theatre or in conversation with his host. Or the well-named dreams of comfort, when a person who likes to prolong his sleep, dreams that he is already up, is washing himself, or is already in school, while as a matter of fact he continues sleeping, hence would rather get up in a dream than in reality. The desire for sleep which we have recognized as a regular part of the dream structure becomes intense in these dreams and appears in them as the actual shaping force of the dream. The wish for sleep properly takes its place beside other great physical desires.

At this point I refer you to a picture by Schwind, from the Schack Gallery in Munich, so that you may see how rightly the artist has conceived the origin of a dream from a dominating situation. It is the *Dream of a Prisoner*,[29] which can have no other subject than his release. It is a very neat stroke that the release should be effected through the window, for the ray of light that awakens the prisoner comes through the same window. The gnomes standing one above the other probably represent the successive positions which he himself had to take in climbing to the height of the window, and I do not think I am mistaken or that I attribute too much preconcerted design to the artist, by noting that the uppermost of the gnomes, who is filing the grating (and so does what the prisoner would like to do) has the features of the prisoner.

In all other dreams except those of children and those of the infantile type, distortion, as we have said, blocks our way. At the outset we cannot ascertain whether they are also wish fulfillments, as we suspect; from their manifest content we cannot determine from what psychic stimulus they derive their origin, and we cannot prove that they also are occupied in doing away with the stimulus and in satisfying it. They must probably be interpreted, that is, translated; their distortion must be annulled; their manifest content replaced by their latent thought before we can judge whether what we have found in children's dreams may claim a universal application for all dreams.

NINTH LECTURE

THE DREAM

The Dream Censor

W E have learned to know the origin, nature and function of the dream from the study of children's dreams. *Dreams are the removal of sleep-disturbing psychic stimuli by way of hallucinated satisfaction.* Of adults' dreams, to be sure, we could explain only one group, what we characterized as dreams of an infantile type. As to the others we know nothing as yet, nor do we understand them. For the present, however, we have obtained a result whose significance we do not wish to underestimate. Every time a dream is completely comprehensible to us, it proves to be an hallucinated wish-fulfillment. This coincidence cannot be accidental, nor is it an unimportant matter.

We conclude, on the basis of various considerations and by analogy to the conception of mistakes, that another type of dream is a distorted substitute for an unknown content and that it must first be led back to that content. Our next task is the investigation and the understanding of this dream distortion.

Dream distortion is the thing which makes the dream seem strange and incomprehensible to us. We want to know several things about it; firstly, whence it comes, its dynamics; secondly, what it does; and finally, how it does it. We can say at this point that dream distortion is the product of the dream work, that is, of the mental functioning of which the dream itself is the conscious symptom. Let us describe the dream work and trace it back to the forces which work upon it.

And now I shall ask you to listen to the following dream. It was recorded by a lady of our profession, and according to her, originated with a highly cultivated and respected lady of advanced age. No analysis of this dream was made. Our informant remarks that to a psychoanalyst it needs no interpretation. The dreamer herself did not interpret it, but she judged and condemned it as if she understood its interpretation. For she said concerning it: "That a woman of fifty should dream such abominable, stupid stuff—a woman who has no other thought, day and night, than to care for her child!"

And now follows the dreams of the "*services of love*." "She goes into Military Hospital No. 1, and says to the sentry at the gate, that she must speak to the chief physician ... (she mentions a name which is not familiar to her), as she wants to offer her service to the hospital. She stresses the word 'service,' so love services. Since she is an old lady he lets her pass after some hesitation. But instead of reaching the chief physician, she finds herself in a large somber room in which there are many officers and army doctors sitting and standing around a long table. She turns with her proposal to a staff doctor who, after a few words, soon understands her. The words of her speech in the dream are, 'I and numerous other women and girls of Vienna are ready for the soldiers, troops, and officers, without distinction....' Here in the dream follows a murmuring. That the idea is, however, correctly understood by those present she sees from the semi-embarrassed, somewhat malicious expressions of the officers. The lady then continues, 'I know that our decision sounds strange, but we are in bitter earnest. The soldier in the field is not asked either whether or not he wants to die.' A moment of painful silence follows. The staff doctor puts his arm around her waist and says, 'Madame, let us assume that it really came to that ...' (murmurs). She withdraws from his arm with the thought, 'They are all alike!' and answers, 'My heavens, I am an old woman, and perhaps will never be confronted with that situation; one consideration, moreover, must be kept in mind: the consideration of age, which prevents an older woman from ... with a very young boy ... (murmurs) ... that would be horrible.' The staff doctor, 'I understand perfectly.' Several officers, among them one who had paid court to her in her youth, laugh loudly, and the lady asks to be conducted to the chief physician, whom she knows, so that everything may be arranged. At this she realizes with great dismay that she does not know his name. The staff officer, nevertheless, very politely and respectfully shows her the way to the second story, up a very narrow winding iron stairway which leads to the upper story directly from the door of the room. In going up she hears an officer say, 'That is a tremendous decision irrespective of whether a woman is young or old; all honor to her!'

"With the feeling that she is merely doing her duty, she goes up an endless staircase."

This dream she repeats twice in the course of a few weeks, with—as the lady notices—quite insignificant and very senseless changes.

This dream corresponds in its structure to a day dream. It has few gaps, and many of its individual points might have been elucidated as to content through inquiry, which, as you know, was omitted. The conspicuous and interesting point for us, however, is that the dream shows several gaps, gaps not of recollection, but of original content. In three places the content is apparently obliterated, the speeches in which these gaps occur are interrupted by murmurs. Since we have performed no analysis, we have, strictly speaking, also no right to make any assertion about the meaning of the dream. Yet there are intimations given from which something may be concluded. For example, the phrase "services of love," and above all the bits of speech which immediately precede the murmurs, demand a completion which can have but one meaning. If we interpolate these, then the phantasy yields as its content the idea that the dreamer is ready, as an act of patriotic duty, to offer her person for the satisfaction of the erotic desires of the army, officers as well as troops. That certainly is exceedingly shocking, it is an impudent libidinous phantasy, but—it does not occur in the dream at all. Just at the point where consistency would demand this confession, there is a vague murmur in the manifest dream, something is lost or suppressed.

I hope you will recognize the inevitability of the conclusion that it is the shocking character of these places in the dream that was the motive for their suppression. Yet where do you find a parallel for this state of affairs? In these times you need not seek far. Take up any political paper and you will find that the text is obliterated here and there, and that in its place shimmers the white of the paper. You know that that is the work of the newspaper censor. In these blank spaces something was printed which was not to the liking of the censorship authorities, and for that reason it was crossed out. You think that it is a pity, that it probably was the most interesting part, it was "the best part."

In other places the censorship did not touch the completed sentence. The author foresaw what parts might be expected to meet with the objection of the censor, and for that reason he softened them by way of prevention, modified them slightly, or contented himself with innuendo and allusion to what really wanted to flow from his pen. Thus the sheet, it is true, has no blank spaces, but from certain circumlocutions and obscurities of expression you will be able to guess that thoughts of the censorship were the restraining motive.

Now let us keep to this parallel. We say that the omitted dream speeches, which were disguised by a murmuring, were also sacrifices to a censorship. We actually speak of a *dream censor* to which we may ascribe a contributing part in the dream distortion. Wherever there are gaps in the manifest dream, it is the fault of the dream censor. Indeed, we should go further, and recognize each time as a manifestation of the dream censor, those places at which a dream element is especially faint, indefinitely and doubtfully recalled among other, more clearly delineated portions. But it is only rarely that this censorship manifests itself so undisguisedly, so naively one may say, as in the example of the dream of the "services of love." Far more frequently the censorship manifests itself according to the second type, through the production of weakenings, innuendoes, allusions instead of direct truthfulness.

For a third type of dream censorship I know of no parallel in the practice of newspaper censorship, yet it is just this type that I can demonstrate by the only dream example which we have so far analyzed. You will remember the dream of the "three bad theatre tickets for one florin and a half." In the latent thoughts of this dream, the element "*precipitately, too soon,*" stood in the foreground. It means: "It was foolish to marry so *early*, it was also foolish to buy theatre tickets so *early*, it was ridiculous of the sister-in-law to spend her money so *hastily*, merely to buy an ornament." Nothing of this central element of the dream thought was evident in the manifest dream. In the latter, going to the theatre and getting the tickets were shoved into the foreground. Through this displacement of the emphasis, this regrouping of the elements of the content, the manifest dream becomes so dissimilar from the latent dream thoughts that no one would suspect the latter behind the former. This displacement of emphasis is a favorite device of the dream distortion and gives the dream that strangeness which makes the dreamer himself unwilling to recognize it as his own production.

Omission, modification, regrouping of the material, these, then, are the effects of the dream censor and the devices of dream distortion. The dream censorship itself is the author, or one of the authors, of the dream distortion whose investigation now occupies us. Modification and rearrangement we are already accustomed to summarize as *displacement*.

After these remarks concerning the effects of the dream censor, let us now turn to their dynamics. I hope you will not consider the expression too anthropomorphically, and picture the dream censor as a severe little manikin who lives in a little brain chamber and there performs his duties; nor should you attempt to localize him too much, to think of a brain center from which his censoring influence emanates, and which would cease with the injury or extirpation of this center. For the present, the term "dream censor" is no more than a very convenient phrase for a dynamic relationship. This phrase does not prevent us from asking by what tendencies such influence is exerted and upon which tendencies it works; nor will we be surprised to discover that we have already encountered the dream censor before, perhaps without recognizing him.

For such was actually the case. You will remember that we had a surprising experience when we began to apply our technique of free association. We then began to feel that some sort of a resistance blocked our efforts to proceed from the dream element to the unconscious element for which the former is the substitute. This resistance, we said, may be of varying strength, enormous at one time, quite negligible at another. In the latter case we need cross only a few intermediate steps in our work of interpretation. But when the resistance is strong, then we must go through a long chain of associations, are taken far afield and must overcome all the difficulties which present themselves as critical objections to the association technique. What we met with in the work of interpretation, we must now bring into the dream work as the dream censor. The resistance to interpretation is nothing but the objectivation of the dream censor. The latter proves to us that the force of the censor has not spent itself in causing the dream distortion, has not since been extinguished, but that this censorship continues as a permanent institution with the purpose of preserving the distortion. Moreover, just as in the interpretation the strength of the resistance varied with each element, so also the distortion produced by the censor in the same dream is of varying magnitude for each element. If one compares the manifest with the latent dream one sees that certain isolated latent elements have been practically eliminated, others more or less modified, and still others left unchanged, indeed, have perhaps been taken over into the dream content with additional strength.

But we wanted to discover what purposes the censorship serves and against which tendencies it acts. This question, which is fundamental to the understanding of the dream, indeed perhaps to human life, is easily answered if we look over a series of those dreams which have been analyzed. The tendencies which the censorship exercises are those which are recognized by the waking judgment of the dreamer, those with which he feels himself in harmony. You may rest assured that when you reject an accurate interpretation of a dream of your own, you do so with the same motives with which the dream censor works, the motives with which it produces the dream distortion and makes the interpretation necessary. Recall the dream of our fifty-year old lady. Without having interpreted it, she considers her dream abominable, would have been still more outraged if our informant had told her anything about the indubitable meaning; and it is just on account of this condemnation that the shocking spots in her dream were replaced by a murmur.

The tendencies, however, against which the dream censor directs itself, must now be described from the standpoint of this instance. One can say only that these tendencies are of an objectionable nature throughout, that they are shocking from an ethical, aesthetic and social point of view, that they are things one does not dare even to think, or thinks of only with abhorrence. These censored wishes which have attained to a distorted expression in the dream, are above all expressions of a boundless, reckless egoism. And indeed, the personal egooccurs in every dream to play the major part in each of them, even if it can successfully disguise itself in the manifest content. This *sacro egoismo* of the dream is surely not unconnected with the sleep-inducing cessation of psychic activity which consists, it should be noted, in the withdrawal of interest from the entire external world.

The ego which has been freed of all ethical restraints feels itself in accord with all the demands of the sexual striving, with those demands which have long since been condemned by our aesthetic rearing, demands of such a character that they resist all our moral demands for restraint. The pleasure-striving—the libido, as we term it—chooses its objects without inhibitions, and indeed, prefers those that are forbidden. It chooses not only the wife of another, but, above all, those incestuous objects declared sacred by the agreement of mankind—the mother and sister in the man's case, the father and brother in the woman's. Even the dream of our fifty-year old lady is an incestuous one, its libido unmistakably directed toward her son. Desires which we believe to be far from human nature show themselves strong enough to arouse dreams. Hate, too, expends itself without restraint. Revenge and murderous wishes toward those standing closest to the dreamer are not unusual, toward those best beloved in daily life, toward parents, brothers and sisters, toward one's spouse and one's own children. These censored wishes seem to arise from a veritable hell; no censorship seems too harsh to be applied against their waking interpretation.

But do not reproach the dream itself for this evil content. You will not, I am sure, forget that the dream is charged with the harmless, indeed the useful function of guarding sleep from disturbance. This evil content, then, does not lie in the nature of the dream. You know also that there are dreams which can be recognized as the satisfaction of justified wishes and urgent bodily needs. These, to be sure, undergo no dream distortion. They need none. They can satisfy their function without offending the ethical and aesthetic tendencies of the ego. And will you also keep in mind the fact that the amount of dream distortion is proportional to two factors. On the one hand, the worse the censorable wish, the greater the distortion; on the other hand, however, the stricter the censor himself is at any particular time the greater the distortion will be also. A young, strictly reared and prudish girl will, by reason of those factors, disfigure with an inexorable censorship those dream impulses which we physicians, for example, and which the dreamer herself ten years later, would recognize as permissible, harmless, libidinous desires.

Besides, we are far from being at the point where we can allow ourselves to be shocked by the results of our work of interpretation. I think we are not yet quite adept at it; and above all there lies upon us the obligation to secure it against certain attacks. It is not at all difficult to "find a hitch" in it. Our dream interpretations were made on the hypotheses we accepted a little while ago, that the dream has some meaning, that from the hypnotic to the normal sleep one may carry over the idea of the existence at such times of an unconscious psychic activity, and that all associations are predetermined. If we had come to plausible results on the basis of these hypotheses, we would have been justified in concluding that the hypotheses were correct. But what is to be done when the results are what I have just pictured them to be? Then it surely is natural to say, "These results are impossible, foolish, at least very improbable, hence there must have been something wrong with the hypotheses. Either the dream is no psychic phenomenon after all, or there is no such thing as unconscious mental activity in the normal condition, or our technique has a gap in it somewhere. Is that not a simpler and more satisfying conclusion than the abominations which we pretend to have disclosed on the basis of our suppositions?"

Both, I answer. It is a simpler as well as a more satisfying conclusion, but not necessarily more correct for that reason. Let us take our time, the matter is not yet ripe for judgment. Above all we can strengthen the criticism against our dream interpretation still further. That its conclusions are so unpleasant and unpalatable is perhaps of secondary importance. A stronger argument is the fact that the dreamers to whom we ascribe such wish-tendencies from the interpretation of their dreams reject the interpretations most emphatically, and with good reason. "What," says the one, "you want to prove to me by this dream that I begrudged the sums which I spent for my sister's trousseau and my brother's education? But indeed that can't be so. Why I work only for my sister, I have no interest in life but to fulfill my duties toward her, as being the oldest child, I promised our blessed mother I would." Or a woman says of her dream, "You mean to say that I wish my husband were dead! Why, that is simply revolting, nonsense. It isn't only that we have the happiest possible married life, you probably won't believe me when I tell you so, but his death would deprive me of everything else that I own in the world." Or another will tell us, "You mean that I have sensual desires toward my sister? That is ridiculous. I am not in the least fond of her. We don't get along and I haven't exchanged a word with her in years." We might perhaps ignore this sort of thing if the dreamers did not confirm or deny the tendencies ascribed to them; we could say that they are matters which the dreamers do not know about themselves. But that the dreamers should feel the exact opposite of the ascribed wish, and should be able to prove to us the dominance of the opposite tendency—this fact must finally disconcert us. Is it not time to lay aside the whole work of the dream interpretation as something whose results reduce it to absurdity?

By no means; this stronger argument breaks down when we attack it critically. Assuming that there are unconscious tendencies in the psychic life, nothing is proved by the ability of the subject to show that their opposites dominate his conscious life. Perhaps there is room in the psychic life even for antithetical tendencies, for contradictions which exist side by side, yes, possibly it is just the dominance of the one impulse which is the necessary condition for the unconsciousness of its opposite. The first two objections raised against our work hold merely that the results of dream interpretation are not simple, and very unpleasant. In answer to the first of these, one may say that for all your enthusiasm for the simple solution, you cannot thereby solve a single dream problem. To do so you must make up your mind to accept the fact of complicated relationships. And to the second of these objections one may say that you are obviously wrong to use a preference or a dislike as the basis for a scientific judgment. What difference does it make if the results of the dream interpretation seem unpleasant, even embarrassing and disgusting to you? "That doesn't prevent them from existing," as I used to hear my teacher Charcot say in similar cases, when I was a young doctor. One must be humble, one must keep personal preferences and antipathies in the background, if one wishes to discover the realities of the world. If a physicist can prove to you that the organic life of this planet must, within a short period of time, become completely extinct, do you also venture to say to him, "That cannot be so. This prospect is too unpleasant." On the contrary, you will be silent until another physicist proves some error in the assumptions or calculations of the first. If you reject the unpleasant, you are repeating the mechanism of dream construction instead of understanding and mastering it.

Perhaps you will promise to overlook the repulsive character of the censored dream-wishes, and will take refuge in the argument that it is improbable, after all, that so wide a field be given over to the evil in the constitution of man. But does your own experience justify you in saying that? I will not discuss the question of how you may estimate yourselves, but have you found so much good will among your superiors and rivals, so much chivalry among your enemies, so little envy in their company, that you feel yourselves in duty bound to enter a protest against the part played by the evil of egoism in human nature? Are you ignorant of how uncontrolled and undependable the average human being is in all the affairs of sex life? Or do you not know that all the immoralities and excesses of which we dream nightly are crimes committed daily by waking persons? What else does psychoanalysis do here but confirm the old saying of Plato, that the good people are those who content themselves with dreaming what the others, the bad people, really do?

And now turn your attention from the individual case to the great war devastating Europe. Think of the amount of brutality, the cruelty and the lies allowed to spread over the civilized world. Do you really believe that a handful of conscienceless egoists and corruptionists could have succeeded in setting free all these evil spirits, if the millions of followers did not share in the guilt? Do you dare under these circumstances to break a lance for the absence of evil from the psychic constitution of mankind?

You will reproach me with judging the war one-sidedly, you will say that it has also brought forth all that is most beautiful and noble in mankind, its heroic courage, its self-sacrifice, its social feeling. Certainly, but do not at this point allow yourselves to become guilty of the injustice which has so often been perpetrated against psychoanalysis, of reproaching it with denying one thing because it was asserting another. It is not our intention to deny the noble strivings of human nature, nor have we ever done anything to deprecate their value. On the contrary, I show you not only the censored evil dream-wishes, but also the censor which suppresses them and renders them unrecognizable. We dwell on the evil in mankind with greater emphasis only because others deny it, a method whereby the psychic life of mankind does not become better, but merely incomprehensible. When, however, we give up this one-sided ethical estimate, we shall surely be able to find a more accurate formula for the relationship of the evil to the good in human nature.

And thus the matter stands. We need not give up the conclusions to which our labors in dream interpretation lead us even though we must consider those conclusions strange. Perhaps we can approach their understanding later by another path. For the present, let us repeat: dream distortion is a consequence of the censorship practised by accredited tendencies of the ego against those wish-impulses that are in any way shocking, impulses which stir in us nightly during sleep. Why these wish-impulses come just at night, and whence they come—these are questions which will bear considerable investigation.

It would be a mistake, however, to omit to mention, with fitting emphasis, another result of these investigations. The dream wishes which try to disturb our sleep are not known to us, in fact we learn of them first through the dream interpretation. Therefore, they may be described as "at that time" unconscious in the sense above defined. But we can go beyond this and say that they are more than merely "at that time" unconscious. The dreamer to be sure denies their validity, as we have seen in so many cases, even after he has learned of their existence by means of the interpretation. The situation is then repeated which we first encountered in the interpretation of the tongue slip "hiccough" where the toastmaster was outraged and assured us that neither then nor ever before had he been conscious of disrespectful impulse toward his chief. This is repeated with every interpretation of a markedly distorted dream, and for that reason attains a significance for our conception. We are now prepared to conclude that there are processes and tendencies in the psychic life of which one knows nothing at all, has known nothing for some time, might, in fact, perhaps never have known anything. The unconscious thus receives a new meaning for us; the idea of "at present" or "at a specific time" disappears from its conception, for it can also mean *permanently* unconscious, not merely *latent at the time*. Obviously we shall have to learn more of this at another session.

Symbolism in the Dream

W E have discovered that the distortion of dreams, a disturbing element in our work of understanding them, is the result of a censorious activity which is directed against the unacceptable of the unconscious wish-impulses. But, of course, we have not maintained that censorship is the only factor which is to blame for the dream distortion, and we may actually make the discovery in a further study of the dream that other items play a part in this result. That is, even if the dream censorship were eliminated we might not be in a position to understand the dreams; the actual dream still might not be identical with the latent dream thought.

This other item which makes the dream unintelligible, this new addition to dream distortion, we discover by considering a gap in our technique. I have already admitted that for certain elements of the dream, no associations really occur to the person being analyzed. This does not happen so often as the dreamers maintain; in many cases the association can be forced by persistence. But still there are certain instances in which no association is forthcoming, or if forced does not furnish what we expected. When this happens in the course of a psychoanalytic treatment, then a particular meaning may be attached thereto, with which we have nothing to do here. It also occurs, however, in the interpretation of the dreams of a normal person or in interpreting one's own dreams. Once a person is convinced that in these cases no amount of forcing of associations will avail, he will finally make the discovery that the unwished-for contingency occurs regularly in certain dream elements, and he will begin to recognize a new order of things there, where at first he believed he had come across a peculiar exception to our technique.

In this way we are tempted to interpret these silent dream elements ourselves, to undertake their translation by the means at hand. The fact that every time we trust to this substitution we obtain a satisfactory meaning is forced upon us; until we resolve upon this decision the dream remains meaningless, its continuity is broken. The accumulation of many similar cases tends to give the necessary certainty to our first timid attempts.

I am expounding all this in rather a schematic manner, but this is permissible for purposes of instruction, and I am not trying to misstate, but only to simplify matters.

In this manner we derive constant translations for a whole series of dream elements just as constant translations are found in our popular dream books for all the things we dream. But do not forget that in our association technique we never discover constant substitutes for the dream elements.

You will say at once that this road to interpretation appears far more uncertain and open to objection than the former methods of free association. But a further fact is to be taken into consideration. After one has gathered a sufficient number of such constant substitutes empirically, he will say that of his own knowledge he should actually have denied that these items of dream interpretation could really be understood without the associations of the dreamer. The facts that force us to recognize their meaning will appear in the second half of our analysis.

We call such a constant relationship between a dream element and its interpretation *symbolic*. The dream element is itself a *symbol* of the unconscious dream thought. You will remember that previously, when we were investigating the relationship between dream elements and their actuality, I drew three distinctions, viz., that of the part of the whole, that of the allusion, and that of the imagery. I then announced that there was a fourth, but did not name it. This fourth is the symbolic relationship here introduced. Very interesting discussions center about this, and we will now consider them before we express our own particular observations on symbolism. Symbolism is perhaps the most noteworthy chapter of dream study.

In the first place, since symbols are permanent or constant translations, they realize, in a certain measure, the ideal of ancient as well as popular dream interpretation, an ideal which by means of our technique we had left behind. They permit us in certain cases to interpret a dream without questioning the dreamer who, aside from this, has no explanation for the symbol. If the interpreter is acquainted with the customary dream symbols and, in addition, with the dreamer himself, the conditions under which the latter lives and the impressions he received before having the dream, it is often possible to interpret a dream without further information—to translate it "right off the bat." Such a trick flatters the interpreter and impresses the dreamer; it stands out as a pleasurable incident in the usual arduous course of cross-examining the dreamer. But do not be misled. It is not our function to perform tricks. Interpretation based on a knowledge of symbols is not a technique that can replace the associative technique, or even compare with it. It is a supplement to the associative technique, and furnishes the latter merely with transplanted, usable results. But as regards familiarity with the dreamer's psychic situation, you must consider the fact that you are not limited to interpreting the dreams of acquaintances; that as a rule you are not acquainted with the daily occurrences which act as the stimuli for the dreams, and that the associations of the subject furnish you with a knowledge of that very thing we call the psychic situation.

Furthermore, it is very extraordinary, particularly in view of circumstances to be mentioned later, that the most vehement opposition has been voiced against the existence of the symbolic relationship between the dream and the unconscious. Even persons of judgment and position, who have otherwise made great progress in psychoanalysis, have discontinued their support at this point. This is the more remarkable since, in the first place, symbolism is neither peculiar to the dream nor characteristic of it, and since in the second place, symbolism in the dream was not discovered through psychoanalysis, although the latter is not poor otherwise in making startling discoveries. The discoverer of dream symbolism, if we insist on a discovery in modern times, was the philosopher K. A. Scherner (1861). Psychoanalysis affirmed Scherner's discovery and modified it considerably.

Now you will want to know something of the nature of dream symbolism, and to hear some examples. I shall gladly impart to you what I know, but I admit that our knowledge is not so complete as we could desire it to be.

The nature of the symbol relationship is a comparison, but not any desired comparison. One suspects a special prerequisite for this comparison, but is unable to say what it is. Not everything to which we are able to compare an object or an occurrence occurs in the dream as its symbol; on the other hand, the dream does not symbolize anything we may choose, but only specific elements of the dream thought. There are limitations on both sides. It must be admitted that the idea of the symbol cannot be sharply delimited at all times—it mingles with the substitution, dramatization, etc., even approaches the allusion. In one series of symbols the basic comparison is apparent to the senses. On the other hand, there are other symbols which raise the question of where the similarity, the "something intermediate" of this suspected comparison is to be sought. We may discover it by more careful consideration, or it may remain hidden to us. Furthermore, it is extraordinary, if the symbol is a comparison, that this comparison is not revealed by the association, that the dreamer is not acquainted with the comparison, that he makes use of it without knowing of its existence. Indeed, the dreamer does not even care to admit the validity of this comparison when it is pointed out to him. So you see, a symbolic relationship is a comparison of a very special kind, the origin of which is not yet clearly understood by us. Perhaps later we may find references to this unknown factor.

The number of things that find symbolic representation in the dream is not great—the human body as a whole, parents, children, brothers and sisters, birth, death, nakedness and a few others. The only typical, that is, regular representation of the human person as a whole is in the form of a *house*, as was recognized by Scherner who, indeed, wished to credit this symbol with an overwhelming significance which it does not deserve. It occurs in dreams that a person, now lustful, now frightened, climbs down the fronts of houses. Those with entirely smooth walls are men; but those which are provided with projections and balconies to which one can hold on, are women. Parents appear in the dream as *king* and *queen*, or other persons highly respected. The dream in this instance is very pious. It treats children, and brothers and sisters, less tenderly; they are symbolized as *little animals* or *vermin*. Birth is almost regularly represented by some reference to *water*; either one plunges into the water or climbs out of it, or rescues someone from the water, or is himself rescued from it, i.e., there is a mother-relation to the person. Death is replaced in the dream by *taking a journey, riding in a train*; *being dead, by various darksome, timid suggestions*; *nakedness, by clothes* and *uniforms*. You see here how the lines between symbolic and suggestive representation merge one into another.

In contrast to the paucity of this enumeration, it is a striking fact that the objects and subject matter of another sphere are represented by an extraordinarily rich symbolism. This is the sphere of the sexual life, the genitals, the sex processes and sexual intercourse. The great majority of symbols in the dream are sex symbols. A remarkable disproportion results from this fact. The designated subject matters are few, their symbols extraordinarily profuse, so that each of these objects can be expressed by any number of symbols of almost equal value. In the interpretation something is disclosed that arouses universal objection. The symbol interpretations, in contrast to the many-sidedness of the dream representations, are very monotonous—this displeases all who deal with them; but what is one to do?

Since this is the first time in these lectures that we speak of the sexual life, I must tell you the manner in which I intend to handle this theme. Psychoanalysis sees no reason for hiding matters or treating them by innuendo, finds no necessity of being ashamed of dealing with this important subject, believes it is proper and decent to call everything by its correct name, and hopes most effectively in this manner to ward off disturbing or salacious thoughts. The fact that I am talking before a mixed audience can make no difference on this point. Just as there is no special knowledge either for the Delphic oracle or for flappers, so the ladies present among you have, by their appearance in this lecture hall, made it clear that they wish to be considered on the same basis as the men.

The dream has a number of representations for the male genital that may be called symbolic, and in which the similarity of the comparison is, for the most part, very enlightening. In the first place, the holy figure 3 is a symbolical substitute for the entire male genital. The more conspicuous and more interesting part of the genital to both sexes, the male organ, has symbolical substitute in objects of like form, those which are long and upright, such as *sticks, umbrellas, poles, trees,* etc. It is also symbolized by objects that have the characteristic, in common with it, of penetration into the body and consequent injury, hence pointed *weapons* of every type, *knives, daggers, lances, swords,* and in the same manner *firearms, guns, pistols* and the *revolver,* which is so suitable because of its shape. In the troubled dream of the young girl, pursuit by a man with a knife or a firearm plays a big role. This, probably the most frequent dream symbolism, is easily translatable. Easily comprehensible, too, is the substitution for the male member of objects out of which water flows: *faucets, water cans, fountains,* as well as its representation by other objects that have the power of elongation, such as *hanging lamps, collapsible pencils,* etc. That *pencils, quills, nail files, hammers* and other *instruments* are undoubtedly male symbols is a fact connected with a conception of the organ, which likewise is not far to seek.

The extraordinary characteristic of the member of being able to raise itself against the force of gravity, one of the phenomena of erection, leads to symbolic representations by *balloons, aeroplanes,* and more recently, *Zeppelins.* The dream has another far more expressive way of symbolizing erection. It makes the sex organ the essential part of the whole person and pictures the person himself as *flying.* Do not feel disturbed because the dreams of flying, often so beautiful, and which we all have had, must be interpreted as dreams of general sexual excitement, as erection dreams. P. Federn, among the psychoanalytical students, has confirmed this interpretation beyond any doubt, and even Mourly Vold, much praised for his sobriety, who carried on his dream experiments with artificial positions of the arms and legs, and who was really opposed to psychoanalysis—perhaps knew nothing about psychoanalysis—has come to the same conclusion as a result of his research. It is no objection to this conclusion that women may have the same dreams of flying. Remember that our dreams act as wish-fulfillments, and that the wish to be a man is often present in women, consciously or unconsciously. And the fact that it is possible for a woman to realize this wish by the same sensation as a man does, will not mislead anyone acquainted with anatomy. There is a small organ in the genitals of a woman similar to that of the male, and this small organ, the clitoris, even in childhood, and in the years before sexual intercourse, plays the same role as does the large organ of the male.

To the less comprehensible male sex-symbols belong certain *reptiles* and *fish*, notably the famous symbol of the *snake*. Why *hats* and *cloaks* should have been turned to the same use is certainly difficult to discover, but their symbolic meaning leaves no room for doubt. And finally the question may be raised whether possibly the substitution of some other member as a representation for the male organ may not be regarded as symbolic. I believe that one is forced to this conclusion by the context and by the female counterparts.

The female genital is symbolically represented by all those objects which share its peculiarity of enclosing a space capable of being filled by something—viz., by *pits*, *caves*, and *hollows*, by *pitchers* and *bottles*, by *boxes* and *trunks*, *jars*, *cases*, *pockets*, etc. The *ship*, too, belongs in this category. Many symbols represent the womb of the mother rather than the female genital, as *wardrobes*, *stoves*, and primarily a *room*. The room-symbolism is related to the house-symbol, *doors* and *entrances* again become symbolic of the genital opening. But materials, too, are symbols of the woman—*wood*, *paper*, and objects that are made of these materials, such as *tables* and *books*. Of animals, at least the *snail* and *mussel* are unmistakably recognizable as symbols for the female; of parts of the body the *mouth* takes the place of the genital opening, while *churches* and *chapels* are structural symbolisms. As you see, all of these symbols are not equally comprehensible.

The breasts must be included in the genitals, and like the larger hemispheres of the female body are represented by *apples*, *peaches* and *fruits* in general. The pubic hair growth of both sexes appears in the dream as *woods* and *bushes*. The complicated topography of the female genitals accounts for the fact that they are often represented as scenes with *cliffs*, *woods* and *water*, while the imposing mechanism of the male sex apparatus leads to the use of all manner of very complicated *machinery*, difficult to describe.

A noteworthy symbol of the female genital is also the *jewel-casket*; *jewels* and *treasure* are also representatives of the beloved person in the dream; *sweets* frequently occur as representatives of sexual delights. The satisfaction in one's own genital is suggested by all types of *play*, in which may be included *piano-playing*. Exquisite symbolic representations of *onanism* are *sliding* and *coasting* as well as *tearing off a branch*. A particularly remarkable dream symbol is that of having *one's teeth fall out*, or *having them pulled*. Certainly its most immediate interpretation is castration as a punishment for onanism. Special representations for the relations of the sexes are less numerous in the dream than we might have expected from the foregoing. Rhythmic activities, such as *dancing*, *riding* and *climbing* may be mentioned, also harrowing experiences, such as *being run over*. One may include certain *manual activities*, and, of course, *being threatened with weapons*.

You must not imagine that either the use or the translation of these symbols is entirely simple. All manner of unexpected things are continually happening. For example, it seems hardly believable that in these symbolic representations the sex differences are not always sharply distinguished. Many symbols represent a genital in general, regardless of whether male or female, e.g., the *little child*, the *small son* or *daughter*. It sometimes occurs that a predominantly male symbol is used for a female genital, or vice versa. This is not understood until one has acquired an insight into the development of the sexual representations of mankind. In many instances this double meaning of symbols may be only apparent; the most striking of the symbols, such as *weapons*, *pockets* and *boxes* are excluded from this bisexual usage.

I should now like to give a summary, from the point of view of the symbols rather than of the thing represented, of the field out of which the sex symbols are for the most part taken, and then to make a few remarks about the symbols which have points in common that are not understood. An obscure symbol of this type is the *hat*, perhaps headdress on the whole, and is usually employed as a male representation, though at times as a female. In the same way the *cloak* represents a man, perhaps not always the genital aspect. You are at liberty to ask, why? The *cravat*, which is suspended and is not worn by women, is an unmistakable male symbol. *White laundry*, all *linen*, in fact, is female. *Dresses*, *uniforms* are, as we have already seen, substitutes for nakedness, for body-formation; the *shoe* or *slipper* is a female genital. *Tables* and *wood* have already been mentioned as puzzling but undoubtedly female symbols. *Ladders*, *ascents*, *steps* in relation to their mounting, are certainly symbols of sexual intercourse. On closer consideration we see that they have the rhythm of walking as a common characteristic; perhaps, too, the heightening of excitement and the shortening of the breath, the higher one mounts.

We have already spoken of *natural scenery* as a representation of the female genitals. *Mountains* and *cliffs* are symbols of the male organ; the *garden* a frequent symbol of the female genitals. *Fruit* does not stand for the child, but for the breasts. *Wild animals* signify sensually aroused persons, or further, base impulses, passions. *Blossoms* and *flowers* represent the female genitals, or more particularly, virginity. Do not forget that the blossoms are really the genitals of the plants.

We already know the *room* as a symbol. The representation may be extended in that the windows, entrances and exits of the room take on the meaning of the body openings. Whether the room is *open* or *closed* is a part of this symbolism, and the *key* that opens it is an unmistakable male symbol.

This is the material of dream symbolism. It is not complete and might be deepened as well as extended. But I am of the opinion it will seem more than enough to you, perhaps will make you reluctant. You will ask, "Do I really live in the midst of sex symbols? Are all the objects that surround me, all the clothes I put on, all the things that I touch, always sex symbols, and nothing else?" There really are sufficient grounds for such questions, and the first is, "Where, in fact, are we to find the meaning of these dream symbols if the dreamer himself can give no information concerning them, or at best can give only incomplete information?"

My answer is: "From many widely different sources, from fairy tales and myths, jokes and farces, from folklore, that is, the knowledge of the customs, usages, sayings and songs of peoples, from the poetic and vulgar language. Everywhere we find the same symbolism and in many of these instances we understand them without further information. If we follow up each of these sources separately we shall find so many parallels to the dream symbolism that we must believe in the correctness of our interpretations."

The human body, we have said, is, according to Scherner, frequently symbolized in the dream by the house. Continuing this representation, the windows, doors and entrances are the entrances into the body cavities, the facades are smooth or provided with balconies and projections to which to hold. The same symbolism is to be found in our daily speech when we greet a good friend as "*old house*" or when we say of someone, "We'll hit him in the *belfry*," or maintain of another that he's not quite right in the *upper story*. In anatomy the body openings are sometimes called the *body-portals*.

The fact that we meet our parents in the dream as imperial or royal persons is at first surprising. But it has its parallel in the fairy tale. Doesn't it begin to dawn upon us that the many fairy tales which begin "Once upon a time there was a *king* and a *queen*" intend nothing else than, "Once there was a *father* and a *mother*?" In our families we refer to our children as *princes*, the eldest as the *crown-prince*. The king usually calls himself the *father of the country*. We playfully designate little children as *worms*, and say, sympathetically, "*poor little worm*."

Let us return to the symbolism of the house. When we use the projections of the house to hold ourselves on to in the dream, are we not reminded of the familiar colloquialism about persons with well-developed breasts: "She has something to *hold onto*"? The folk express this in still another way when it says, "there's lots of *wood in front of her house*"; as though it wished to come to the aid of our interpretation that wood is a feminine, maternal symbol.

In addition to wood there are others. We might not understand how this material has come to be a substitute for the maternal, the feminine. Here our comparison of languages may be helpful. The German word *Holz* (wood) is said to be from the same stem as the Greek word, ὕλη, which means stuff, raw material. This is an example of the case, not entirely unusual, where a general word for material finally is exclusively used for some special material. There is an island in the ocean, known by the name of Madeira. The Portuguese gave it this name at the time of its discovery because it was at that time entirely covered with forests, for in the language of the Portuguese, Madeira means *wood*. You will recognize, however, that Madeira, is nothing else than the slightly changed Latin word *materia* which again has the general meaning of *material* Material is derived from *mater*, mother. The material out of which something is made, is at the same time its mother-part. In the symbolic use of wood for woman, mother, this ancient conception still lives.

Birth is regularly expressed in dreams by some connection with water; one plunges into the water, or comes out of the water, which means one gives birth to, or is born. Now let us not forget that this symbol may refer in two ways to the truths of evolutionary history. Not alone have all land-mammals, including the ancestors of man, developed out of water animals—this is the ultimate fact—but every single mammal, every human being, lived the first part of his existence in the water—namely, lived in the body of his mother as an embryo in the amniotic fluid and came out of the water at the time of his birth. I do not wish to maintain that the dreamer knows this, on the contrary I hold that he does not have to know. The dreamer very likely knows some things because of the fact that he was told about them in his childhood, and for that very reason I maintain that this knowledge has played no part in the construction of his symbols. He was told in childhood that the stork brought him—but where did it get him? Out of a lake, out of the well—again, out of the water. One of my patients to whom such information had been given, a little count, disappeared for a whole afternoon. Finally he was discovered lying at the edge of the palace lake, his little face bent above the water and earnestly peering into it to see if he could not see the little children at the bottom.

In the myths of the birth of the hero, which O. Rank submitted to comparative examination,—the oldest is that of King Sargon of Agade, about 2800 B.C.—exposure in the water and rescue from water play a predominating role. Rank has recognized that these are representations of birth, analogous to those customary in dreams. When a person in his dream rescues another from the water, the latter becomes his mother, or just plainly mother; in the myth a person who rescues a child out of the water professes herself as the real mother of the child. In a well-known joke the intelligent Jewish boy is asked who was the mother of Moses. He answered without hesitation, the Princess. But no, he is told, she only took him out of the water. "That's what *she says*," is his reply, and thereby he shows that he has found the correct interpretation of the myth.

Leaving on a trip represents death in the dream. Likewise it is the custom in the nursery when a child asks where someone who has died, and whom he misses, may be, to say to him that the absent one has taken a trip. Again I should like to deny the truth of the belief that the dream symbol originates in this evasion used for the benefit of children. The poet makes use of the same symbol when he speaks of the Hereafter as "that undiscovered bourne from which no *traveler* returns." Even in everyday speech it is customary to refer to the last journey. Every person acquainted with ancient rite knows how seriously, for example, the Egyptians considered the portrayal of a journey to the land of the dead. There still exist many copies of the "death book" which was given to the mummy for this journey as a sort of Baedeker. Since the burial places have been separated from the living quarters, the last journey of the dead person has become a reality.

In the same manner the genital symbolism is just as little peculiar to the dream alone. Every one of you has perhaps at some time or other been so unkind as to call some woman an "*old casket*" without perhaps being aware that he was using a genital symbol. In the New Testament one may read "Woman is a weak *vessel*." The Holy Scriptures of the Jews, so nearly poetic in their style, are filled with sex-symbolic expressions which have not always been correctly understood, and the true construction of which, in the *Song of Songs*, for example, has led to many misunderstandings. In the later Hebraic literature the representation of woman as a house, the door taking the place of the sex opening, is very widespread. The man complains, for instance, when he discovers a lack of virginity, that he has found *the door open*. The symbol of the table for woman is also known to this literature. The woman says of her husband, "I set the table for him, *but he upset it*." Lame children are supposed to result from the fact that the man has *overturned the table*. I take these examples from a work by L. Levy of Brünn, *The Sexual Symbolism of the Bible and the Talmud*.

That ships, too, represent women in dreams is a belief derived from the etymologists, who maintain "ship" was originally the name of an earthen vessel and is the same word as *Schaff* (to create). The Greek myth of Periander of Corinth and his wife Melissa is proof that the stove or oven is a woman, and a womb. When, according to Herodotus, the tyrant entreated the shade of his beloved wife, whom, however, he had murdered in a fit of jealousy, for some sign of its identity, the deceased identified herself by the reminder that he, *Periander, had thrust his bread into a cold oven*, as a disguise for an occurrence that could have been known to no other person. In the *Anthropophyteia* published by F. S. Krauss, an indispensable source book for everything that has to do with the sex life of nations, we read that in a certain German region it is commonly said of a woman who has just been delivered of a child, "*Her oven has caved in*." The making of a fire and everything connected therewith is filled through and through with sex symbolism. The flame is always the male genital, the fireplace, the hearth, is the womb of the woman.

If you have often wondered why it is that landscapes are so often used to represent the female genitals in the dream, then let the mythologist teach you the role Mother Earth has played in the symbolisms and cults of ancient times. You may be tempted to say that a room represents a woman in the dream because of the German colloquialism which uses the term *Frauenzimmer* instead of *Frau*, in other words, it substitutes for the human person the idea of that room that is set aside for her exclusive use. In like manner we speak of the *Sublime Porte*, and mean the Sultan and his government; furthermore, the name of the ancient Egyptian ruler,

Pharaoh, means nothing other than "great court room." (In the ancient Orient the court yards between the double gates of the town were the gathering places of the people, in the same manner as the market place was in the classical world.) What I mean is, this derivation is far too superficial. It seems more probable to me that the room, as the space surrounding man, came to be the symbol of woman. We have seen that the house is used in such a representation; from mythology and poetry we may take the *city, fortress, palace, citadel,* as further symbols of woman. The question may easily be decided by the dreams of those persons who do not speak German and do not understand it. In the last few years my patients have been predominantly foreign-language speaking, and I think I can recall that in their dreams as well the room represents woman, even where they had no analogous usages in their languages. There are still other signs which show that the symbolization is not limited by the bounds of language, a fact that even the old dream investigator, Schubert (1862) maintained. Since none of my dreamers were totally ignorant of German I must leave this differentiation to those psychoanalysts who can gather examples in other lands where the people speak but one language.

Among the symbol-representations of the male genital there is scarcely one that does not recur in jokes or in vulgar or poetical usage, especially among the old classical poets. Not alone do those symbols commonly met with in dreams appeal here, but also new ones, e.g., the working materials of various performances, foremost of which is the incantation. Furthermore, we approach in the symbolic representation of the male a very extended and much discussed province, which we shall avoid for economic reasons. I should like to make a few remarks, however, about one of the unclassified symbols—the figure 3. Whether or not this figure derives its holiness from its symbolic meaning may remain undecided. But it appears certain that many objects which occur in nature as three-part things derive their use as coats-of-arms and emblems from such symbolic meaning, e.g., the clover, likewise the three-part French lily, (fleur-de-lys), and the extraordinary coats-of-arms of two such widely separated islands as Sicily and the Isle of Man, where the Triskeles (three partly bended knees, emerging from a central point) are merely said to be the portrayal in a different form of the male genitals. Copies of the male member were used in antiquity as the most powerful charms (*Apotropaea*) against evil influences, and this is connected with the fact that the lucky amulets of our own time may one and all be recognized as genital or sex-symbols. Let us study such a collection, worn in the form of little silver pendants: the four-leaf clover, a pig, a mushroom, a horse-shoe, a ladder, a chimney-sweep. The four-leaf clover, it seems, has usurped the place of the three-leaf clover, which is really more suitable as a symbol; the pig is an ancient symbol of fertility; the mushroom is an unquestionable penis symbol—there are mushrooms that derive their systematic names from their unmistakable similarity to the male member (Phallus impudicus); the horseshoe recalls the contour of the female genital opening; and the chimney sweep who carries a ladder belongs in this company because he carries on that trade with which the sex-intercourse is vulgarly compared (*cf.* the *Anthropophyteia*). We have already become acquainted with his ladder as a sex symbol in the dream; the German usage is helpful here, it shows us how the verb "to mount"[30] is made use of in an exquisite sexual sense. We use the expressions "*to run after women*," which literally translated would be "*to climb after women*," and "*an old climber*."[31] In French, where "*step*" is "*la marche*" we find that the analogous expression for a man about town is "*un vieux marcheur*." It is apparently not unknown in this connection that the sexual intercourse of many of the larger animals requires a mounting, *a climbing upon* the female.

The tearing off of a branch as the symbolic representation of onanism is not alone in keeping with the vulgar representation of the fact of onanism, but has far-reaching mythological parallels. Especially noteworthy, however, is the representation of onanism, or rather the punishment therefor, castration, by the falling out or pulling out of teeth, because there is a parallel in folk-lore which is probably known to the fewest dreamers. It does not seem at all questionable to me that the practice of circumcision common among so many peoples is an equivalent and a substitute for castration. And now we are informed that in Australia certain primitive tribes practice circumcision as a rite of puberty (the ceremony in honor of the boy's coming of age), while others, living quite near, have substituted for this act the striking out of a tooth.

I end my exposition with these examples. They are only examples. We know more about these matters, and you may well imagine how much richer and how much more interesting such a collection would appear if made, not by amateurs like ourselves, but by real experts in mythology, anthropology, philology and folk-lore. We are compelled to draw a few conclusions which cannot be exhaustive, but which give us much food for thought.

In the first place, we are faced by the fact that the dreamer has at his disposal a symbolic means of expression of which he is unconscious while awake, and does not recognize when he sees. That is as remarkable as if you should make the discovery that your chambermaid understands Sanskrit, although you know she was born in a Bohemian village and never learned the language. It is not easy to harmonize this fact with our psychological views. We can only say that the dreamer's knowledge of symbolism is unconscious, that it is a part of his unconscious mental life. We make no progress with this assumption. Until now it was only necessary to admit of unconscious impulses, those about which one knew nothing, either for a period of time or at all times. But now we deal with something more; indeed, with unknown knowledge, with thought relationships, comparisons between unlike objects which lead to this, that one constant may be substituted for another. These comparisons are not made anew each time, but they lie ready, they are complete for all time. That is to be concluded from the fact of their agreement in different persons, agreement despite differences in language.

But whence comes the knowledge of these symbol-relationships? The usages of language cover only a small part of them. The dreamer is for the most part unacquainted with the numerous parallels from other sources; we ourselves must first laboriously gather them together.

Secondly, these symbolic representations are peculiar neither to the dreamer nor to the dream work by means of which they become expressed. We have learned that mythology and fairy-tales make use of the same symbolism, as well as do the people in their sayings and songs, the ordinary language of every day, and poetic phantasy. The field of symbolism is an extraordinarily large one, and dream symbolism is but a small part thereof. It is not even expedient to approach the whole problem from the dream side. Many of the symbols that are used in other places do not occur in the dream at all, or at best only very seldom. Many of the dream symbols are to be found in other fields only very rarely, as you have seen. One gets the impression that he is here confronted with an ancient but no longer existent method of expression, of which various phases, however, continue in different fields, one here, one there, a third, perhaps in a slightly altered form, in several fields. I am reminded of the phantasy of an interesting mental defective, who had imagined a fundamental language, of which all these symbolic representations were the remains.

Thirdly, you must have noticed that symbolism in these other fields is by no means sex symbolism solely, while in the dream the symbols are used almost entirely to express sexual objects and processes. Nor is this easily explained. Is it possible that symbols originally sexual in their meaning later came to have other uses, and that this was the reason perhaps for the weakening of the symbolic representation to one of another nature? These questions are admittedly unanswerable if one has dealt only with dream-symbolism. One can only adhere to the supposition that there is an especially intimate connection between true symbols and things sexual.

An important indication of this has been given us recently. A philologist, H. Sperber (Upsala) who works independently of psychoanalysis, advanced the theory that sexual needs have played the largest part in the origin and development of languages. The first sounds served as means of communication, and called the sexual partner; the further development of the roots of speech accompanied the performance of the primitive man's work. This work was communal and progressed to the accompaniment of rhythmically repeated word sounds. In that way a sexual interest was transferred to the work. The primitive man made work acceptable at the same time that he used it as an equivalent and substitute for sex-activity. The word thus called forth by the common labor had two meanings, designating the sex-act as well as the equivalent labor-activity. In time the word became disassociated from its sexual significance and became fixed on this work. Generations later the same thing happened to a new word that once had sexual significance and came to be used for a new type of work. In this manner a number of word-roots were formed, all of sexual origin, and all of which had lost their sexual significance. If the description sketched here approximates the truth, it opens up the possibility for an understanding of the dream symbolism. We can understand how it is that in the dream, which preserves something of these most ancient conditions, there are so extraordinarily many symbols for the sexual, and why, in general, weapons and implements always stand for the male, materials and things manufactured, for the female. Symbolic relationships would be the remnants of the old word-identity; things which once were called by the same names as the genitals can now appear in the dream as symbols for them.

From our parallels to dream symbolization you may also learn to appreciate what is the character of psychoanalysis which makes it a subject of general interest, which is true of neither psychology nor psychiatry. Psychoanalytic work connects with so many other scientific subjects, the investigation of which promises the most pertinent discoveries, with mythology, with folk-lore, with racial psychology and with religion. You will understand how a journal can have grown on psychoanalytic soil, the sole purpose of which is the furtherance of these relationships. This is the *Imago* founded in 1912 and edited by Hanns Sachs and Otto Rank. In all of these relations, psychoanalysis is first and foremost the giving, less often the receiving, part. Indeed it derives benefit from the fact that its unusual teachings are substantiated by their recurrence in other fields, but on the whole it is psychoanalysis that provides the technical procedure and the point of view, the use of which will prove fruitful in those other fields. The psychic life of the human individual provides us, upon psychoanalytic investigation, with explanations with which we are able to solve many riddles in the life of humanity, or at least show these riddles in their proper light.

Furthermore, I have not even told you under what conditions we are able to get the deepest insight into that suppositious "fundamental language," or from which field we gain the most information. So long as you do not know this you cannot appreciate the entire significance of the subject. This field is the neurotic, its materials, the symptoms and other expressions of the nervous patient, for the explanation and treatment of which psychoanalysis was devised.

My fourth point of view returns to our premise and connects up with our prescribed course. We said, even if there were no such thing as dream censorship, the dream would still be hard to understand, for we would then be confronted with the task of translating the symbol-language of the dream into the thought of our waking hours. Symbolism is a second and independent item of dream distortion, in addition to dream censorship. It is not a far cry to suppose that it is convenient for the dream censorship to make use of symbolism since both lead to the same end, to making the dream strange and incomprehensible.

Whether or not in the further study of the dream we shall hit upon a new item that influences dream distortion, remains to be seen. I should not like to leave the subject of dream symbolism without once more touching upon the curious fact that it arouses such strong opposition in the case of educated persons, in spite of the fact that symbolism in myth, religion, art and speech is undoubtedly so prevalent. Is not this again because of its relationship to sexuality?

ELEVENTH LECTURE

THE DREAM

The Dream-Work

IF you have mastered dream censorship and symbolic representation, you are, to be sure, not yet adept in dream distortion, but you are nevertheless in a position to understand most dreams. For this you employ two mutually supplementary methods, call up the associations of the dreamer until you have penetrated from the substitute to the actual, and from your own knowledge supply the meaning for the symbol. Later we shall discuss certain uncertainties which show themselves in this process.

We are now in a position to resume work which we attempted, with very insufficient means at an earlier stage, when we studied the relation between the manifest dream elements and their latent actualities, and in so doing established four such main relationships: that of a part of the whole, that of approach or allusion, the symbolic relationship and plastic word representation. We shall now attempt the same on a larger scale, by comparing the manifest dream content as a whole, with the latent dream which we found by interpretation.

I hope you will never again confuse these two. If you have achieved this, you have probably accomplished more in the understanding of the dream than the majority of the readers of my *Interpretation of Dreams*. Let me remind you once more that this process, which changes the latent into the manifest dream, is called *dream-work*. Work which proceeds in the opposite direction, from the manifest dream to the latent, is our *work of interpretation*. The work of interpretation attempts to undo the dream-work. Infantile dreams that are recognized as evident wish fulfillments nevertheless have undergone some dream-work, namely, the transformation of the wish into reality, and generally, too, of thoughts into visual pictures. Here we need no interpretation, but only a retracing of these transformations. Whatever dream-work has been added to other dreams, we call *dream distortion*, and this can be annulled by our work of interpretation.

The comparison of many dream interpretations has rendered it possible for me to give you a coherent representation of what the dream-work does with the material of the latent dream. I beg of you, however, not to expect to understand too much of this. It is a piece of description that should be listened to with calm attention.

The first process of the dream-work is *condensation*. By this we understand that the manifest dream has a smaller content than the latent one, that is, it is a sort of abbreviated translation of the latter. Condensation may occasionally be absent, but as a rule it is present, often to a very high degree. The opposite is never true, that is, it never occurs that the manifest dream is more extensive in scope and content than the latent. Condensation occurs in the following ways: 1. Certain latent elements are entirely omitted; 2. only a fragment of the many complexes of the latent dream is carried over into the manifest dream; 3. latent elements that have something in common are collected for the manifest dream and are fused into a whole.

If you wish, you may reserve the term "condensation" for this last process alone. Its effects are particularly easy to demonstrate. From your own dreams you will doubtless recall the fusion of several persons into one. Such a compound person probably looks like A., is dressed like B., does something that one remembers of C., but in spite of this one is conscious that he is really D. By means of this compound formation something common to all four people is especially emphasized. One can make a compound formation of events and of places in the same way as of people, provided always that the single events and localities have something in common which the latent dream emphasizes. It is a sort of new and fleeting concept of formation, with the common element as its kernel. This jumble of details that has been fused together regularly results in a vague indistinct picture, as though you had taken several pictures on the same film.

The shaping of such compound formations must be of great importance to the dream-work, for we can prove, (by the choice of a verbal expression for a thought, for instance) that the common elements mentioned above are purposely manufactured where they originally do not exist. We have already become acquainted with such condensation and compound formations; they played an important part in the origin of certain cases of slips of the tongue. You recall the young man who wished to *inscort* a woman. Furthermore, there are jokes whose technique may be traced to such a condensation. But entirely aside from this, one may maintain that this appearance of something quite unknown in the dream finds its counterpart in many of the creations of our imagination which fuse together component parts that do not belong together in experience, as for example the centaurs, and the fabulous animals of old mythology or of Boecklin's pictures. For creative imagination can invent nothing new whatsoever, it can only put together certain details normally alien to one another. The peculiar thing, however, about the procedure of the dream-work is the following: The material at the disposal of the dream-work consists of thoughts, thoughts which may be offensive and unacceptable, but which are nevertheless correctly formed and expressed. These thoughts are transformed into something else by the dream-work, and it is remarkable and incomprehensible that this translation, this rendering, as it were, into another script or language, employs the methods of condensation and combination. For a translation usually strives to respect the discriminations expressed in the text, and to differentiate similar things. The dream-work, on the contrary, tries to fuse two different thoughts by looking, just as the joke does, for an ambiguous word which shall act as a connecting link between the two thoughts. One need not attempt to understand this feature of the case at once, but it may become significant for the conception of the dream-work.

Although condensation renders the dream opaque, one does not get the impression that it is an effect of dream censorship. One prefers to trace it back to mechanical or economic conditions; but censorship undoubtedly has a share in the process.

The results of condensation may be quite extraordinary. With its help, it becomes possible at times to collect quite unrelated latent thought processes into one manifest dream, so that one can arrive at an apparently adequate interpretation, and at the same time conceive a possible further interpretation.

The consequence of condensation for the relation between latent and manifest dreams is the fact that no simple relations can exist between the elements of the one and the other. A manifest element corresponds simultaneously to several latent ones, and vice versa, a latent element may partake of several manifest ones, an interlacing, as it were. In the interpretation of the dream it also becomes evident that the associations to a single element do not necessarily follow one another in orderly sequence. Often we must wait until the entire dream is interpreted.

Dream-work therefore accomplishes a very unusual sort of transcription of dream thoughts, not a translation word for word, or sign for sign, not a selection according to a set rule, as if all the consonants of a word were given and the vowels omitted; nor is it what we might call substitution, namely, the choice of one element to take the place of several others. It is something very different and much more complicated.

The second process of the dream-work is *displacement*. Fortunately we are already prepared for this, since we know that it is entirely the work of dream censorship. The two evidences of this are firstly, that a latent element is not replaced by one of its constituent parts but by something further removed from it, that is, by a sort of allusion; secondly, that the psychic accent is transferred from an important element to another that is unimportant, so that the dream centers elsewhere and seems strange.

Substitution by allusion is known to our conscious thinking also, but with a difference. In conscious thinking the allusion must be easily intelligible, and the substitute must bear a relation to the actual content. Jokes, too, often make use of allusion; they let the condition of content associations slide and replace it by unusual external associations, such as resemblances in sound, ambiguity of words, etc. They retain, however, the condition of intelligibility; the joke would lose all its effect if the allusion could not be traced back to the actual without any effort whatsoever. The allusion of displacement has freed itself of both these limitations. Its connection with the element which it replaces is most external and remote, is unintelligible for this reason, and if it is retraced, its interpretation gives the impression of an unsuccessful joke or of a forced, far-fetched explanation. For the dream censor has only then accomplished its purpose, when it has made the path of return from the allusion to the original undiscoverable.

The displacement of emphasis is unheard of as a means of expressing thoughts. In conscious thinking we occasionally admit it to gain a comic effect. I can probably give you an idea of the confusion which this produces by reminding you of the story of the blacksmith who had committed a capital crime. The court decided that the penalty for the crime must be paid, but since he was the only blacksmith in the village and therefore indispensable, while there were three tailors, one of the latter was hung in his stead.

The third process of the dream-work is the most interesting from a psychological point of view. It consists of the *translation* of thoughts into visual images. Let us bear in mind that by no means all dream thoughts undergo this translation; many of them retain their form and appear in the manifest dream also as thought or consciousness; moreover, visual images are not the only form into which thoughts are translated. They are, however, the foundation of the dream fabric; this part of the dream work is, as we already know, the second most constant, and for single dream elements we have already learned to know "plastic word representation."

It is evident that this process is not simple. In order to get an idea of its difficulties you must pretend that you have undertaken the task of replacing a political editorial in a newspaper by a series of illustrations, that you have suffered an atavistic return from the use of the alphabet to ideographic writing. Whatever persons or concrete events occur in this article you will be able to replace easily by pictures, perhaps to your advantage, but you will meet with difficulties in the representation of all abstract words and all parts of speech denoting thought relationships, such as particles, conjunctions, etc. With the abstract words you could use all sorts of artifices. You will, for instance, try to change the text of the article into different words which may sound unusual, but whose components will be more concrete and more adapted to representation. You will then recall that most abstract words were concrete before their meaning paled, and will therefore go back to the original concrete significance of these words as often as possible, and so you will be glad to learn that you can represent the "possession" of an object by the actual physical straddling of it.[32] The dream work does the same thing. Under such circumstances you can hardly demand accuracy of representation. You will also have to allow the dream-work to replace an element that is as hard to depict as for instance, broken faith, by another kind of rupture, a broken leg.[33] In this way you will be able to smooth away to some extent the crudity of imagery when the latter is endeavoring to replace word expression.

In the representation of parts of speech that denote thought relations, such as *because*, *therefore*, *but*, etc., you have no such aids; these constituent parts of the text will therefore be lost in your translation into images. In the same way, the dream-work resolves the content of the dream thought into its raw material of objects and activities. You may be satisfied if the possibility is vouchsafed you to suggest certain relations, not representable in themselves, in a more detailed elaboration of the image. In quite the same way the dream-work succeeds in expressing much of the content of the latent dream thought in the formal peculiarities of the manifest dream, in its clearness or vagueness, in its division into several parts, etc. The number of fragmentary dreams into which the dream is divided corresponds as a rule to the number of main themes, of thought sequences in the latent dream; a short preliminary dream often stands as an introduction or a motivation to the complementary dream which follows; a subordinate clause in dream thought is represented in the manifest dream as an interpolated change of scene, etc. The form of the dream is itself, therefore, by no means without significance and challenges interpretation. Different dreams of the same night often have the same meaning, and testify to an increasing effort to control a stimulus of growing urgency. In a single dream a particularly troublesome element may be represented by "duplicates," that is, by numerous symbols.

By continually comparing dream thought with the manifest dream that replaces it, we learn all sorts of things for which we were not prepared, as for instance, the fact that even the nonsense and absurdity of the dream have meaning. Yes, on this point the opposition between the medical and psychoanalytic conception of the dream reaches a climax not previously achieved. According to the former, the dream is senseless because the dreaming psychic activity has lost all power of critical judgment; according to our theory, on the other hand, the dream becomes senseless, whenever a critical judgment, contained in the dream thought, wishes to express the opinion: "It is nonsense." The dream which you all know, about the visit to the theatre (three tickets 1 Fl. 50 Kr.) is a good example of this. The opinion expressed here is: "It was *nonsense* to marry so early."

In the same way, we discover in interpretation what is the significance of the doubts and uncertainties so often expressed by the dreamer as to whether a certain element really occurred in the dream; whether it was this or something else. As a rule these doubts and uncertainties correspond to nothing in the latent dream thought; they are occasioned throughout by the working of the dream censor and are equivalent to an unsuccessful attempt at suppression.

One of the most surprising discoveries is the manner in which the dream-work deals with those things which are opposed to one another in the latent dream. We already know that agreements in the latent material are expressed in the manifest dream by condensations. Now oppositions are treated in exactly the same way as agreements and are, with special preference, expressed by the same manifest element. An element in a manifest dream, capable of having an opposite, may therefore represent itself as well as its opposite, or may do both simultaneously; only the context can determine which translation is to be chosen. It must follow from this that the particle "no" cannot be represented in the dream, at least not unambiguously.

The development of languages furnishes us with a welcome analogy for this surprising behavior on the part of the dream work. Many scholars who do research work in languages have maintained that in the oldest languages opposites—such as strong, weak; light, dark; big, little—were expressed by the same root word. (*The Contradictory Sense of Primitive Words.*) In old Egyptian, *ken* originally meant both strong and weak. In conversation, misunderstanding in the use of such ambiguous words was avoided by the tone of voice and by accompanying gestures, in writing by the addition of so-called determinatives, that is, by a picture that was itself not meant to be expressed. Accordingly, if ken meant strong, the picture of an erect little man was placed after the alphabetical signs, if *ken*, *weak*, was meant, the picture of a cowering man followed. Only later, by slight modifications of the original word, were two designations developed for the opposites which it denoted. In this way, from *ken* meaning both strong and weak, there was derived a *ken*, strong, and a *ken*, weak. It is said that not only the most primitive languages in their last developmental stage, but also the more recent ones, even the living tongues of to-day have retained abundant remains of this primitive opposite meaning. Let me give you a few illustrations of this taken from C. Abel (1884).

In Latin there are still such words of double meaning:

altus—high, deep, and *sacer*, sacred, accursed.

As examples of modifications of the same root, I cite:

clamare—to scream, *clam*—quiet, still, secret;

siccus—dry, *succus*—juice.

And from the German:

Stimme—voice, *stumm*—dumb.

The comparison of related tongues yields a wealth of examples:

English: *lock*; German: *Loch*—hole, *Lücke*—gap.

English: *cleave*; German: *kleben*—to stick, to adhere.

The English *without*, is to-day used to mean "not with"; that "with" had the connotation of deprivation as well as that of apportioning, is apparent from the compounds: *withdraw*, *withhold*. The German *wieder*, again, closely resembles this.

Another peculiarity of dream-work finds it prototype in the development of language. It occurred in ancient Egyptian as well as in other later languages that the sequence of sounds of the words was transposed to denote the same fundamental idea. The following are examples from English and German:

Topf—pot; *boat*—tub; *hurry*—*Ruhe* (rest, quiet).

Balken (beam)—*Kloben* (mallet)—*club*.

From the Latin and the German:

capere (to seize)—*packen* (to seize, to grasp).

Inversions such as occur here in the single word are effected in a very different way by the dream-work. We already know the inversion of the sense, substitution by the opposite. Besides there are inversions of situations, of relations between two people, and so in dreams we are in a sort of topsy-turvy world. In a dream it is frequently the rabbit that shoots the hunter. Further inversion occurs in the sequence of events, so that in the dream the cause is placed after the effect. It is like a performance in a third-rate theatre, where the hero falls before the shot which kills him is fired from the wings. Or there are dreams in which the whole sequence of the elements is inverted, so that in the interpretation one must take the last first, and the first last, in order to obtain a meaning. You will recall from our study of dream symbolism that to go or fall into the water means the same as to come out of it, namely, to give birth to, or to be born, and that mounting stairs or a ladder means the same as going down. The advantage that dream distortions may gain from such freedom of representation, is unmistakable.

These features of the dream-work may be called *archaic*. They are connected with ancient systems of expression, ancient languages and literatures, and involve the same difficulties which we shall deal with later in a critical connection.

Now for some other aspects of the matter. In the dream-work it is plainly a question of translating the latent thoughts, expressed in words, into psychic images, in the main, of a visual kind. Now our thoughts were developed from such psychic images; their first material and the steps which led up to them were psychic impressions, or to be more exact, the memory images of these psychic impressions. Only later were words attached to these and then combined into thoughts. The dream-work therefore puts the thoughts through a *regressive* treatment, that is, one that retraces the steps in their development. In this regression, all that has been added to the thoughts as a new contribution in the course of the development of the memory pictures must fall away.

This, then, is the dream-work. In view of the processes that we have discovered about it, our interest in the manifest dream was forced into the background. I shall, however, devote a few remarks to the latter, since it is after all the only thing that is positively known to us.

It is natural that the manifest dream should lose its importance for us. It must be a matter of indifference to us whether it is well composed or resolved into a series of disconnected single images. Even when its exterior seems to be significant, we know that it has been developed by means of dream distortion and may have as little organic connection with the inner content of the dream as the facade of an Italian church has with its structure and ground plan. At other times this facade of the dream, too, has its significance, in that it reproduces with little or no distortion an important part of the latent dream thought. But we cannot know this before we have put the dream through a process of interpretation and reached a decision as to what amount of distortion has taken place. A similar doubt prevails when two elements in the dream seem to have been brought into close relations to one another. This may be a valuable hint, suggesting that we may join together those manifest thoughts which correspond to the elements in the latent dream; yet at other times we are convinced that what belongs together in thought has been torn apart in the dream.

As a general rule we must refrain from trying to explain one part of the manifest dream by another, as if the dream were coherently conceived and pragmatically represented. At the most it is comparable to a Breccian stone, produced by the fusion of various minerals in such a way that the markings it shows are entirely different from those of the original mineral constituents. There is actually a part of the dream-work, the so-called *secondary treatment*, whose function it is to develop something unified, something approximately coherent from the final products of the dream-work. In so doing the material is often arranged in an entirely misleading sense and insertions are made wherever it seems necessary.

On the other hand, we must not over-estimate the dream-work, nor attribute too much to it. The processes which we have enumerated tell the full tale of its functioning; beyond condensing, displacing, representing plastically, and then subjecting the whole to a secondary treatment, it can do nothing. Whatever of judgment, of criticism, of surprise, and of deduction are to be found in the dream are not products of the dream-work and are only very seldom signs of afterthoughts about the dream, but are generally parts of the latent dream thought, which have passed over into the manifest dream, more or less modified and adapted to the context. In the matter of composing speeches, the dream-work can also do nothing. Except for a few examples, the speeches in the dream are imitations and combinations of speeches heard or made by oneself during the day, and which have been introduced into the latent thought, either as material or as stimuli for the dream. Neither can the dream pose problems; when these are found in the dream, they are in the main combinations of numbers, semblances of examples that are quite absurd or merely copies of problems in the latent dream thought. Under these conditions it is not surprising that the interest which has attached itself to the dream-work is soon deflected from it to the latent dream thoughts which are revealed in more or less distorted form in the manifest dream. It is not justifiable, however, to have this change go so far that in a theoretical consideration one regularly substitutes the latent dream thought for the dream itself, and maintains of the latter what can hold only for the former. It is odd that the results of psychoanalysis should be misused for such an exchange. "Dream" can mean nothing but the result of the dream-work, that is, the *form* into which the latent dream thoughts have been translated by the dream-work.

Dream-work is a process of a very peculiar sort, the like of which has hitherto not been discovered in psychic life. These condensations, displacements, regressive translations of thoughts into pictures, are new discoveries which richly repay our efforts in the field of psychoanalysis. You will realize from the parallel to the dream-work, what connections psychoanalytic studies will reveal with other fields, especially with the development of speech and thought. You can only surmise the further significance of these connections when you hear that the mechanism of the dream structure is the model for the origin of neurotic symptoms.

I know too that we cannot as yet estimate the entire contribution that this work has made to psychology. We shall only indicate the new proofs that have been given of the existence of unconscious psychic acts—for such are the latent dream thoughts—and the unexpectedly wide approach to the understanding of the unconscious psychic life that dream interpretation opens up to us.

The time has probably come, however, to illustrate separately, by various little examples of dreams, the connected facts for which you have been prepared.

TWELFTH LECTURE

THE DREAM

Analysis of Sample Dreams

$\mathbf{I}$HOPE you will not be disappointed if I again lay before you excerpts from dream analyses instead of inviting you to participate in the interpretation of a beautiful long dream. You will say that after so much preparation you ought to have this right, and that after the successful interpretation of so many thousands of dreams it should long ago have become possible to assemble a collection of excellent dream samples with which we could demonstrate all our assertions concerning dream-work and dream thoughts. Yes, but the difficulties which stand in the way of the fulfillment of your wish are too many.

First of all, I must confess to you that no one practices dream interpretation as his main occupation. When does one interpret dreams? Occasionally one can occupy himself with the dream of some friend, without any special purpose, or else he may work with his own dreams for a time in order to school himself in psychoanalytic method; most often, however, one deals with the dreams of nervous individuals who are undergoing analytic treatment. These latter dreams are excellent material, and in no way inferior to those of normal persons, but one is forced by the technique of the treatment to subordinate dream analysis to therapeutic aims and to pass over a large number of dreams after having derived something from them that is of use in the treatment. Many dreams we meet with during the treatment are, as a matter of fact, impossible of complete analysis. Since they spring from the total mass of psychic material which is still unknown to us, their understanding becomes possible only after the completion of the cure. Besides, to tell you such dreams would necessitate the disclosure of all the secrets concerning a neurosis. That will not do for us, since we have taken the dream as preparation for the study of the neuroses.

I know you would gladly leave this material, and would prefer to hear the dreams of healthy persons, or your own dreams explained. But that is impossible because of the content of these dreams. One can expose neither himself, nor another whose confidence he has won, so inconsiderately as would result from a thorough interpretation of his dreams—which, as you already know, refer to the most intimate things of his personality. In addition to this difficulty, caused by the nature of the material, there is another that must be considered when communicating a dream. You know the dream seems strange even to the dreamer himself, let alone to one who does not know the dreamer. Our literature is not poor in good and detailed dream analyses. I myself have published some in connection with case histories. Perhaps the best example of a dream interpretation is the one published by O. Rank, being two related dreams of a young girl, covering about two pages of print, the analysis covering seventy-six pages. I would need about a whole semester in order to take you through such a task. If we select a longer or more markedly distorted dream, we have to make so many explanations, we must make use of so many free associations and recollections, must go into so many bypaths, that a lecture on the subject would be entirely unsatisfactory and inconclusive. So I must ask you to be content with what is more easily obtained, with the recital of small bits of dreams of neurotic persons, in which we may be able to recognize this or that isolated fact. Dream symbols are the most easily demonstrable, and after them, certain peculiarities of regressive dream representations.[34] I shall tell you why I considered each of the following dreams worthy of communication.

1. A dream, consisting of only two brief pictures: "*The dreamer's uncle is smoking a cigarette, although it is Saturday. A woman caresses him as though he were her child.*"

In commenting on the first picture, the dreamer (a Jew) remarks that his uncle is a pious man who never did, and never would do, anything so sinful as smoking on the Sabbath. As to the woman of the second picture, he has no free associations other than his mother. These two pictures or thoughts should obviously be brought into connection with each other, but how? Since he expressly rules out the reality of his uncle's action, then it is natural to interpolate an "if." "*If* my uncle, that pious man, should smoke a cigarette on Saturday, then I could also permit my mother's caresses." This obviously means that the mother's caresses are prohibited, in the same manner as is smoking on Saturday, to a pious Jew. You will recall, I told you that all relations between the dream thoughts disappear in the dream-work, that these relations are broken up into their raw material, and that it is the task of interpretation to re-interpolate the omitted connections.

2. Through my publications on dreams I have become, in certain respects, the public consultant on matters pertaining to dreams, and for many years I have been receiving communications from the most varied sources, in which dreams are related to me or presented to me for my judgment. I am of course grateful to all those persons who include with the story of the dream, enough material to make an interpretation possible, or who give such an interpretation themselves. It is in this category that the following dream belongs, the dream of a Munich physician in the year 1910. I select it because it goes to show how impossible of understanding a dream generally is before the dreamer has given us what information he has about it. I suspect that at bottom you consider the ideal dream interpretation that in which one simply inserts the meaning of the symbols, and would like to lay aside the technique of free association to the dream elements. I wish to disabuse your minds of this harmful error.

"On July 13, 1910, toward morning, I dreamed *that I was bicycling down a street in Tübingen, when a brown Dachshund tore after me and caught me by the heel. A bit further on I get off, seat myself on a step, and begin to beat the beast, which has clenched its teeth tight. (I feel no discomfort from the biting or the whole scene.) Two elderly ladies are sitting opposite me and watching me with grins on their faces. Then I wake up and, as so often happens to me, the whole dream becomes perfectly clear to me in this moment of transition to the waking state."*

Symbols are of little use in this case. The dreamer, however, informs us, "I lately fell in love with a girl, just from seeing her on the street, but had no means of becoming acquainted with her. The most pleasant means might have been the Dachshund, since I am a great lover of animals, and also felt that the girl was in sympathy with this characteristic." He also adds that he repeatedly interfered in the fights of scuffling dogs with great dexterity and frequently to the great amazement of the spectators. Thus we learn that the girl, who pleased him, was always accompanied by this particular dog. This girl, however, was disregarded in the manifest dream, and there remained only the dog which he associates with her. Perhaps the elderly ladies who simpered at him took the place of the girl. The remainder of what he tells us is not enough to explain this point. Riding a bicycle in the dream is a direct repetition of the remembered situation. He had never met the girl with the dog except when he was on his bicycle.

3. When anyone has lost a loved one, he produces dreams of a special sort for a long time afterward, dreams in which the knowledge of death enters into the most remarkable compromises with the desire to have the deceased alive again. At one time the deceased is dead and yet continues to live on because he does not know that he is dead, and would die completely only if he knew it; at another time he is half dead and half alive, and each of these conditions has its particular signs. One cannot simply label these dreams nonsense, for to come to life again is no more impossible in the dream than, for example, it is in the fairy story, in which it occurs as a very frequent fate. As far as I have been able to analyze such dreams, I have always found them to be capable of a sensible solution, but that the pious wish to recall the deceased to life goes about expressing itself by the oddest methods. Let me tell you such a dream, which seems queer and senseless enough, and analysis of which will show you many of the points for which you have been prepared by our theoretical discussions. The dream is that of a man who had lost his father many years previously.

"Father is dead, but has been exhumed and looks badly. He goes on living, and the dreamer does everything to prevent him from noticing that fact." Then the dream goes on to other things, apparently irrelevant.

The father is dead, that we know. That he was exhumed is not really true, nor is the truth of the rest of the dream important. But the dreamer tells us that when he came back from his father's funeral, one of his teeth began to ache. He wanted to treat this tooth according to the Jewish precept, "If thy tooth offend thee, pluck it out," and betook himself to the dentist. But the latter said, "One does not simply pull a tooth out, one must have patience with it. I shall inject something to kill the nerve. Come again in three days and then I will take it out."

"This 'taking it out'," says the dreamer suddenly, "is the exhuming."

Is the dreamer right? It does not correspond exactly, only approximately, for the tooth is not taken out, but something that has died off is taken out of it. But after our other experiences we are probably safe in believing that the dream work is capable of such inaccuracies. It appears that the dreamer condensed, fused into one, his dead father and the tooth that was killed but retained. No wonder then, that in the manifest dream something senseless results, for it is impossible for everything that is said of the tooth to fit the father. What is it that serves as something intermediate between tooth and father and makes this condensation possible?

This interpretation must be correct, however, for the dreamer says that he is acquainted with the saying that when one dreams of losing a tooth it means that one is going to lose a member of his family.

We know that this popular interpretation is incorrect, or at least is correct only in a scurrilous sense. For that reason it is all the more surprising to find this theme thus touched upon in the background of other portions of the dream content.

Without any further urging, the dreamer now begins to tell of his father's illness and death as well as of his relations with him. The father was sick a long time, and his care and treatment cost him, the son, much money. And yet it was never too much for him, he never grew impatient, never wished it might end soon. He boasts of his true Jewish piety toward his father, of rigid adherence to the Jewish precepts. But are you not struck by a contradiction in the thoughts of the dream? He had identified tooth with father. As to the tooth he wanted to follow the Jewish precept that carries out its own judgment, "pull it out if it causes pain and annoyance." He had also been anxious to follow the precept of the law with regard to his father, which in this case, however, tells him to disregard trouble and expense, to take all the burdens upon himself and to let no hostile intent arise toward the object which causes the pain. Would not the agreement be far more compelling if he had really developed feelings toward his father similar to those about his sick tooth; that is, had he wished that a speedy death should put an end to that superfluous, painful and expensive existence?

I do not doubt that this was really his attitude toward his father during the latter's extended illness, and that his boastful assurances of filial piety were intended to distract his attention from these recollections. Under such circumstances, the death-wish directed toward the parent generally becomes active, and disguises itself in phrases of sympathetic consideration such as, "It would really be a blessed release for him." But note well that we have here overcome an obstacle in the latent dream thoughts themselves. The first part of these thoughts was surely unconscious only temporarily, that is to say, during the dream-work, while the inimical feelings toward the father might have been permanently unconscious, dating perhaps from childhood, occasionally slipping into consciousness, shyly and in disguise, during his father's illness. We can assert this with even greater certainty of other latent thoughts which have made unmistakable contributions to the dream content. To be sure, none of these inimical feelings toward the father can be discovered in the dream. But when we search a childhood history for the root of such enmity toward the father, we recollect that fear of the father arises because the latter, even in the earliest years, opposes the boy's sex activities, just as he is ordinarily forced to oppose them again, after puberty, for social motives. This relation to the father applies also to our dreamer; there had been mixed with his love for him much respect and fear, having its source in early sex intimidation.

From the onanism complex we can now explain the other parts of the manifest dream. "*He looks badly*" does, to be sure, allude to another remark of the dentist, that it looks badly to have a tooth missing in that place; but at the same time it refers to the "looking badly" by which the young man betrayed, or feared to betray, his excessive sexual activity during puberty. It was not without lightening his own heart that the dreamer transposed the bad looks from himself to his father in the manifest content, an inversion of the dream work with which you are familiar. "*He goes on living since then,*" disguises itself with the wish to have him alive again as well as with the promise of the dentist that the tooth will be preserved. A very subtle phrase, however, is the following: "The dreamer does everything *to prevent him* (*the father*) *from noticing the fact,*" a phrase calculated to lead us to conclude that he is dead. Yet the only meaningful conclusion is again drawn from the onanism complex, where it is a matter of course for the young man to do everything in order to hide his sex life from his father. Remember, in conclusion, that we were constantly forced to interpret the so-called tooth-ache dreams as dreams dealing with the subject of onanism and the punishment that is feared.

You now see how this incomprehensible dream came into being, by the creation of a remarkable and misleading condensation, by the fact that all the ideas emerge from the midst of the latent thought process, and by the creation of ambiguous substitute formations for the most hidden and, at the time, most remote of these thoughts.

4. We have tried repeatedly to understand those prosaic and banal dreams which have nothing foolish or repulsive about them, but which cause us to ask: "Why do we dream such unimportant stuff?" So I shall give you a new example of this kind, three dreams belonging together, all of which were dreamed in the same night by a young woman.

(*a*). "*She it going through the hall of her house and strikes her head against the low-hanging chandelier, so that her head bleeds.*"

She has no reminiscence to contribute, nothing that really happened. The information she gives leads in quite another direction. "You know how badly my hair is falling out. Mother said to me yesterday, 'My child, if it goes on like this, you will have a head like the cheek of a buttock.'" Thus the head here stands for the other part of the body. We can understand the chandelier symbolically without other help; all objects that can be lengthened are symbols of the male organ. Thus the dream deals with a bleeding at the lower end of the body, which results from its collision with the male organ. This might still be ambiguous; her further associations show that it has to do with her belief that menstrual bleeding results from sexual intercourse with a man, a bit of sexual theory believed by many immature girls.

(*b*). "*She sees a deep hole in the vineyard which she knows was made by pulling out a tree.*" Herewith her remark that "*she misses the tree.*" She means that she did not see the tree in the dream, but the same phrase serves to express another thought which symbolic interpretation makes completely certain. The dream deals with another bit of the infantile sex theory, namely, with the belief that girls originally had the same genitals as boys and that the later conformation resulted from castration (pulling out of a tree).

(*c*). "*She is standing in front of the drawer of her writing table, with which she is so familiar that she knows immediately if anybody has been through it.*" The writing-table drawer, like every drawer, chest, or box, stands for the female genital. She knows that one can recognize from the genital the signs of sexual intercourse (and, as she thinks, even of any contact at all) and she has long been afraid of such a conviction. I believe that the accent in all these dreams is to be laid upon the idea of *knowing*. She is reminded of the time of her childish sexual investigations, the results of which made her quite proud at the time.

5. Again a little bit of symbolism. But this time I must first describe the psychic situation in a short preface. A man who spent the night with a woman describes his partner as one of those motherly natures whose desire for a child irresistibly breaks through during intercourse. The circumstances of their meeting, however, necessitated a precaution whereby the fertilizing discharge of semen is kept away from the womb. Upon awaking after this night, the woman tells the following dream:

"*An officer with a red cap follows her on the street. She flees from him, runs up the staircase, and he follows after her. Breathlessly she reaches her apartment and slams and locks the door behind her. He remains outside and as she looks through a peephole she sees him sitting outside on a bench and weeping.*"

You undoubtedly recognize in the pursuit by an officer with a red cap, and the breathless stair climbing, the representation of the sexual act. The fact that the dreamer locks herself in against the pursuer may serve as an example of that inversion which is so frequently used in dreams, for in reality it was the man who withdrew before the completion of the act. In the same way her grief has been transposed to the partner, it is he who weeps in the dream, whereby the discharge of the semen is also indicated.

You must surely have heard that in psychoanalysis it is always maintained that all dreams have a sexual meaning. Now you yourselves are in a position to form a judgment as to the incorrectness of this reproach. You have become acquainted with the wish-fulfillment dreams, which deal with the satisfying of the plainest needs, of hunger, of thirst, of longing for freedom, the dreams of convenience and of impatience and likewise the purely covetous and egoistic dreams. But that the markedly distorted dreams preponderantly—though again not exclusively—give expression to sex wishes, is a fact you may certainly keep in mind as one of the results of psychoanalytical research.

6. I have a special motive for piling up examples of the use of symbols in dreams. At our first meeting I complained of how hard it is, when lecturing on psychoanalysis, to demonstrate the facts in order to awaken conviction; and you very probably have come to agree with me since then. But the various assertions of psychoanalysis are so closely linked that one's conviction can easily extend from

one point to a larger part of the whole. We might say of psychoanalysis that if we give it our little finger it promptly demands the whole hand. Anyone who was convinced by the explanation of errors can no longer logically disbelieve in all the rest of psychoanalysis. A second equally accessible point of approach is furnished by dream symbolism. I shall give you a dream, already published, of a peasant woman, whose husband is a watchman and who has certainly never heard anything about dream symbolism and psychoanalysis. You may then judge for yourselves whether its explanation with the help of sex symbols can be called arbitrary and forced.

"Then someone broke into her house and she called in fright for a watchman. But the latter had gone companionably into a church together with two 'beauties.' A number of steps led up to the church. Behind the church was a hill, and on its crest a thick forest. The watchman was fitted out with a helmet, gorget and a cloak. He had a full brown beard. The two were going along peacefully with the watchman, had sack-like aprons bound around their hips. There was a path from the church to the hill. This was overgrown on both sides with grass and underbrush that kept getting thicker and that became a regular forest on the crest of the hill."

You will recognize the symbols without any difficulty. The male genital is represented by a trinity of persons, the female by a landscape with a chapel, hill and forest. Again you encounter steps as the symbol of the sexual act. That which is called a hill in the dream has the same name in anatomy, namely, *mons veneris*, the mount of Venus.

7. I have another dream which can be solved by means of inserting symbols, a dream that is remarkable and convincing because the dreamer himself translated all the symbols, even though he had had no preliminary knowledge of dream interpretation. This situation is very unusual and the conditions essential to its occurrence are not clearly known.

"He is going for a walk with his father in some place which must be the Prater,[35] for one can see the rotunda and before it a smaller building to which is anchored a captive balloon, which, however, seems fairly slack. His father asks him what all that is for; he wonders at it himself but explains it to his father. Then they come to a courtyard in which there lies spread out a big sheet of metal. His father wants to break off a big piece of it for himself but first looks about him to see if anyone might see him. He says to him that all he needs to do is to tell the inspector and then he can take some without more ado. There are steps leading from this courtyard down into a pit, the walls of which are upholstered with some soft material rather like a leather arm chair. At the end of this pit is a longish platform and then a new pit begins...."

The dreamer himself interprets as follows: "The rotunda is my genital, the balloon in front of it is my penis, of whose slackness I have been complaining." Thus one may translate in more detail, that the rotunda is the posterior—a part of the body which the child regularly considers as part of the genital—while the smaller building before it is the scrotum. In the dream his father asks him what all that is for; that is to say, he asks the object and function of the genitals. It is easy to turn this situation around so that the dreamer is the one who does the asking. Since no such questioning of the father ever took place in real life, we must think of the thought of this dream as a wish or consider it in the light of a supposition, "If I had asked father for sexual enlightenment." We will find the continuation of this idea in another place shortly.

The courtyard, in which the sheet metal lies spread out, is not to be considered primarily as symbolical but refers to the father's place of business. For reasons of discretion I have substituted the "sheet metal" for another material with which the father deals, without changing anything in the literal wording of the dream. The dreamer entered his father's business and took great offense at the rather dubious practices upon which the profits depended to a large extent. For this reason the continuation of the above idea of the dream might be expressed as "if I had asked him, he would only have deceived me as he deceives his customers." The dreamer himself gives us the second meaning of "breaking off the metal," which serves to represent the commercial dishonesty. He says it means masturbation. Not only have we long since become familiar with this symbol, but the fact also is in agreement. The secrecy of masturbation is expressed by means of its opposite—"It can be safely done openly." Again our expectations are fulfilled by the fact that masturbatory activity is referred to as the father's, just as the questioning was in the first scene of the dream. Upon being questioned he immediately gives the interpretation of the pit as the vagina on account of the soft upholstering of its walls. I will add arbitrarily that the "going down" like the more usual "going up" is meant to describe the sexual intercourse in the vagina.

Such details as the fact that the first pit ends in a platform and then a new one begins, he explains himself as having been taken from his own history. He practiced intercourse for a while, then gave it up on account of inhibitions, and now hopes to be able to resume it as a result of the treatment.

8. The two following dreams are those of a foreigner, of very polygamous tendencies, and I give them to you as proof for the claim that one's ego appears in every dream, even in those in which it is disguised in the manifest content. The trunks in the dream are a symbol for woman.

(*a*). "*He is to take a trip, his luggage is placed on a carriage to be taken to the station, and there are many trunks piled up, among which are two big black ones like sample trunks. He says, consolingly, to someone, 'Well, they are only going as far as the station with us.'*"

In reality he does travel with a great deal of luggage, but he also brings many tales of women with him when he comes for treatment. The two black trunks stand for two dark women who play the chief part in his life at present. One of them wanted to travel to Vienna after him, but he telegraphed her not to, upon my advice.

(*b*). A scene at the customs house: "*A fellow traveler opens his trunk and says indifferently while puffing a cigarette, 'There's nothing in here.' The customs official seems to believe him but delves into the trunk once more and finds something particularly forbidden. The traveler then says resignedly, 'Well, there's no help for it.'"*

He himself is the traveler, I the customs official. Though otherwise very frank in his confessions, he has on this occasion tried to conceal from me a new relationship which he had struck up with a lady whom he was justified in believing that I knew. The painful situation of being convicted of this is transposed into a strange person so that he himself apparently is not present in the dream.

9. The following is an example of a symbol which I have not yet mentioned:

"He meets his sister in company with two friends who are themselves sisters. He extends his hand to both of them but not to his sister."

This is no allusion to a real occurrence. His thoughts instead lead him back to a time when his observations made him wonder why a girl's breasts develop so late. The two sisters, therefore, are the breasts. He would have liked to touch them if only it had not been his sister.

10. Let me add an example of a symbol of death in a dream:

"He is walking with two persons whose name he knows but has forgotten. By the time he is awake, over a very high, steep iron bridge. Suddenly the two people are gone and he sees a ghostly man with a cap, and clad in white. He asks this man whether he is the telegraph messenger.... No. Or is he a coachman? No. Then he goes on," and even in the dream he is in great fear. After waking he continues the dream by a phantasy in which the iron bridge suddenly breaks, and he plunges into the abyss.

When the dreamer emphasizes the fact that certain individuals in a dream are unknown, that he has forgotten their names, they are generally persons standing in very close relationship to the dreamer. This dreamer has two sisters; if it be true, as his dream indicates, that he wished these two dead, then it would only be justice if the fear of death fell upon him for so doing. In connection with the telegraph messenger he remarks that such people always bring bad news. Judged by his uniform he might also have been the lamp-lighter, who, however, also extinguishes the lamps—in other words, as the spirit of death extinguishes the flame of life. The coachman reminds him of Uhland's poem of King Karl's ocean voyage and also of a dangerous lake trip with two companions in which he played the role of the king in the poem. In connection with the iron bridge he remembers a recent accident and the stupid saying "Life is a suspension bridge."

11. The following may serve as another example of the representation of death in a dream: *"An unknown man leaves a black bordered visiting card for him."*

12. The following dream will interest you for several reasons, though it is one arising from a neurotic condition among other things:

"He is traveling in a train. The train stops in an open field. He thinks it means that there is going to be an accident, that he must save himself, and he goes through all the compartments of the train and strikes dead everyone whom he meets, conductors, engine drivers, etc."

In connection with this he tells a story that one of his friends told him. An insane man was being transported in a private compartment in a certain place in Italy, but through some mistake another traveler was put in the same compartment. The insane man murdered his fellow passenger. Thus he identifies himself with this insane person and bases his right so to do upon a compulsive idea which was then torturing him, namely, he must "do away with all persons who knew of his failings." But then he himself finds a better motivation which gave rise to the dream. The day before, in the theatre, he again saw the girl whom he had expected to marry but whom he had left because she had given him cause for jealousy. With a capacity for intense jealousy such as he has, he would really be insane if he married. In other words, he considers her so untrustworthy that out of jealousy he would have to strike dead all the persons who stood in his way. Going through a series of rooms, of compartments in this case, we have already learned to recognize as the symbol of marriage (the opposite of monogamy).

In connection with the train stopping in the open country and his fear of an accident, he tells the following: Once, when he was traveling in a train and it came to a sudden stop outside of a station, a young lady in the compartment remarked that perhaps there was going to be a collision, and that in that case the best precaution would be to pull one's legs up. But this "legs up" had also played a role in the many walks and excursions into the open which he had taken with the girl in that happy period in their first love. Thus it is a new argument for the idea that he would have to be crazy in order to marry her now. But from my knowledge of the situation I can assume with certainty that the wish to be as crazy as that nevertheless exists in him.

THIRTEENTH LECTURE

THE DREAM

Archaic Remnants and Infantilism in the Dream

LET us revert to our conclusion that the dream-work, under the influence of the dream censorship, transforms the latent dream thoughts into some other form of expression. The latent thoughts are no other than the conscious thoughts known to us in our waking hours; the new mode of expression is incomprehensible to us because of its many-sided features. We have said it extends back to conditions of our intellectual development which we have long progressed beyond, to the language of pictures, the symbol-representations, perhaps to those conditions which were in force before the development of our language of thought. So we called the mode of expression of the dream-work the archaic or regressive.

You may conclude that as a result of the deeper study of the dream-work we gain valuable information about the rather unknown beginnings of our intellectual development. I trust this will be true, but this work has not, up to the present time, been undertaken. The antiquity into which the dream-work carries us back is of a double aspect, firstly, the individual antiquity, childhood; and, secondly (in so far as every individual in his childhood lives over again in some more or less abbreviated manner the entire development of the human race), also this antiquity, the philogenetic. That we shall be able to differentiate which part of the latent psychic proceeding has its source in the individual, and which part in the philogenetic antiquity is not improbable. In this connection it appears to me, for example, that the symbolic relations which the individual has never learned are ground for the belief that they should be regarded as a philogenetic inheritance.

However, this is not the only archaic characteristic of the dream. You probably all know from your own experiences the peculiar amnesia, that is, loss of memory, concerning childhood. I mean the fact that the first years, to the fifth, sixth or eighth, have not left the same traces in our memory as have later experiences. One meets with individual persons, to be sure, who can boast of a continuous memory from the very beginning to the present day, but the other condition, that of a gap in the memory, is far more frequent. I believe we have not laid enough stress on this fact. The child is able to speak well at the age of two, it soon shows that it can become adjusted to the most complicated psychic situations, and makes remarks which years later are retold to it, but which it has itself entirely forgotten. Besides, the memory in the early years is more facile, because it is less burdened than in later years. Nor is there any reason for considering the memory-function as a particularly high or difficult psychic performance; in fact, the contrary is true, and you can find a good memory in persons who stand very low intellectually.

As a second peculiarity closely related to the first, I must point out that certain well-preserved memories, for the most part formatively experienced, stand forth in this memory-void which surrounds the first years of childhood and do not justify this hypothesis. Our memory deals selectively with its later materials, with impressions which come to us in later life. It retains the important and discards the unimportant. This is not true of the retained childhood memories. They do not bespeak necessarily important experiences of childhood, not even such as from the viewpoint of the child need appear of importance. They are often so banal and intrinsically so meaningless that we ask ourselves in wonder why just these details have escaped being forgotten. I once endeavored to approach the riddle of childhood amnesia and the interrupted memory remnants with the help of analysis, and I arrived at the conclusion that in the case of the child, too, only the important has remained in the memory, except that by means of the process of condensation already known to you, and especially by means of distortion, the important is represented in the memory by something that appears unimportant. For this reason I have called these childhood memories "disguise-memories," memories used to conceal; by means of careful analysis one is able to develop out of them everything that is forgotten.

In psychoanalytic treatment we are regularly called upon to fill out the infantile memory gaps, and in so far as the cure is to any degree successful, we are able again to bring to light the content of the childhood years thus clouded in forgetfulness. These impressions have never really been forgotten, they have only been inaccessible, latent, have belonged to the unconscious. But sometimes they bob up out of the unconscious spontaneously, and, as a matter of fact, this is what happens in dreams. It is apparent that the dream life knows how to find the entrance to these latent, infantile experiences. Beautiful examples of this occur in literature, and I myself can present such an example. I once dreamed in a certain connection of a person who must have performed some service for me, and whom I clearly saw. He was a one-eyed man, short in stature, stout, his head deeply sunk into his neck. I concluded from the content that he was a physician. Luckily I was able to ask my mother, who was still living, how the physician in my birth-place, which I left when I was three years old, looked, and I learned from her that he had one eye, was short and stout, with his head sunk into his neck, and also learned at what forgotten mishap he had been of service to me. This control over the forgotten material of childhood years is, then, a further archaic tendency of the dream.

The same information may be made use of in another of the puzzles that have presented themselves to us. You will recall how astonished people were when we came to the conclusion that the stimuli which gave rise to dreams were extremely bad and licentious sexual desires which have made dream-censorship and dream-distortion necessary. After we have interpreted such a dream for the dreamer and he, in the most favorable circumstances does not attack the interpretation itself, he almost always asks the question whence such a wish comes, since it seems foreign to him and he feels conscious of just the opposite sensations. We need not hesitate to point out this origin. These evil wish-impulses have their origin in the past, often in a past which is not too far away. It can be shown that at one time they were known and conscious, even if they no longer are so. The woman, whose dream is interpreted to mean that she would like to see her seventeen-year old daughter dead, discovers under our guidance that she in fact at one time entertained this wish. The child is the fruit of an unhappy marriage, which early ended in a separation. Once, while the child was still in the womb, and after a tense scene with her husband, she beat her body with her fists in a fit of anger, in order to kill the child. How many mothers who to-day love their children tenderly, perhaps too tenderly, received them unwillingly, and at the time wished that the life within them would not develop further; indeed, translated this wish into various actions, happily harmless. The later death-wish against some loved one, which seems so strange, also has its origin in early phases of the relationship to that person.

The father, the interpretation of whose dream shows that he wishes for the death of his eldest and favorite child, must be reminded of the fact that at one time this wish was no stranger to him. While the child was still a suckling, this man, who was unhappy in his choice of a wife, often thought that if the little being that meant nothing to him would die, he would again be free, and would make better use of his freedom. A like origin may be found for a large number of similar hate impulses; they are recollections of something that belonged to the past, were once conscious and played their parts in the psychic life. You will wish to conclude therefrom that such wishes and such dreams cannot occur if such changes in the relationship to a person have not taken place; if such relationship was always of the same character. I am ready to admit this, only wish to warn you that you are to take into consideration not the exact terms of the dream, but the meaning thereof according to its interpretation. It may happen that the manifest dream of the death of some loved person has only made use of some frightful mask, that it really means something entirely different, or that the loved person serves as a concealing substitute for some other.

But the same circumstances will call forth another, more difficult question. You say: "Granted this death wish was present at some time or other, and is substantiated by memory, yet this is no explanation. It is long outlived, to-day it can be present only in the unconscious and as an empty, emotionless memory, but not as a strong impulse. Why should it be recalled by the dream at all!" This question is justified. The attempt to answer it would lead us far afield and necessitate taking up a position in one of the most important points of dream study. But I must remain within the bounds of our discussion and practice restraint. Prepare yourselves for the temporary abstention. Let us be satisfied with the circumstantial proof that this outlived wish can be shown to act as a dream stimulator and let us continue the investigation to see whether or not other evil wishes admit of the same derivation out of the past.

Let us continue with the removal or death-wish which most frequently can be traced back to the unbounded egoism of the dreamer. Such a wish can very often be shown to be the inciting cause of the dream. As often as someone has been in our way in life—and how often must this happen in the complicated relationships of life—the dream is ready to do away with him, be he father, mother, brother, sister, spouse, etc. We have wondered sufficiently over this evil tendency of human nature, and certainly were not predisposed to accept the authenticity of this result of dream interpretation without question. After it has once been suggested to us to seek the origin of such wishes in the past, we disclose immediately the period of the individual past in which such egoism and such wish-impulses, even as directed against those closest to the dreamer, are no longer strangers. It is just in these first years of childhood which later are hidden by amnesia, that this egoism frequently shows itself in most extreme form, and from which regular but clear tendencies thereto, or real remnants thereof, show themselves. For the child loves itself first, and later learns to love others, to sacrifice something of its ego for another. Even those persons whom the child seems to love from the very beginning, it loves at the outset because it has need of them, cannot do without them, in others words, out of egoistical motives. Not until later does the love impulse become independent of egoism. *In brief, egoism has taught the child to love.*

In this connection it is instructive to compare the child's regard for his brothers and sisters with that which he has for his parents. The little child does not necessarily love his brothers and sisters, often, obviously, he does not love them at all. There is no doubt that in them he hates his rivals and it is known how frequently this attitude continues for many years until maturity, and even beyond, without interruption. Often enough this attitude is superseded by a more tender feeling, or rather let us say glossed over, but the hostile feeling appears regularly to have been the earlier. It is most noticeable in children of from two and one-half to four or five years of age, when a new little brother or sister arrives. The latter is usually received in a far from friendly manner. Expressions such as "I don't want him! Let the stork take him away again," are very usual. Subsequently every opportunity is made use of to disparage the new arrival, and even attempts to do him bodily harm, direct attacks, are not unheard of. If the difference in age is less, the child learns of the existence of the rival with intense psychic activity, and accommodates himself to the new situation. If the difference in age is greater, the new child may awaken certain sympathies as an interesting object, as a sort of living doll, and if the difference is eight years or more, motherly impulses, especially in the case of girls, may come into play. But to be truthful, when we disclose in a dream the wish for the death of a mother or sister we need seldom find it puzzling and may trace its origin easily to early childhood, often enough, also, to the propinquity of later years.

Probably no nurseries are free from mighty conflicts among the inhabitants. The motives are rivalry for the love of the parents, articles owned in common, the room itself. The hostile impulses are called forth by older as well as younger brothers and sisters. I believe it was Bernard Shaw who said: "If there is anyone who hates a young English lady more than does her mother, it is her elder sister." There is something about this saying, however, that arouses our antipathy. We can, at a pinch, understand hatred of brothers and sisters, and rivalry among them, but how may feelings of hatred force their way into the relationship between daughter and mother, parents and children?

This relationship is without doubt the more favorable, even when looked at from the viewpoint of the child. This is in accord with our expectation; we find it much more offensive for love between parents and children to be lacking than for love between brothers and sisters. We have, so to speak, made something holy in the first instance which in the other case we permitted to remain profane. But daily observation can show us how frequently the feelings between parents and their grown children fail to come up to the ideal established by society, how much enmity exists and would find expression did not accumulations of piety and of tender impulse hold them back. The motives for this are everywhere known and disclose a tendency to separate those of the same sex, daughter from mother, father from son. The daughter finds in her mother the authority that hems in her will and that is entrusted with the task of causing her to carry out the abstention from sexual liberty which society demands; in certain cases also she is the rival who objects to being displaced. The same type of thing occurs in a more glaring manner between father and son. To the son the father is the embodiment of every social restriction, borne with such great opposition; the father bars the way to freedom of will, to early sexual satisfaction, and where there is family property held in common, to the enjoyment thereof. Impatient waiting for the death of the father grows to heights approximating tragedy in the case of a successor to the throne. Less strained is the relationship between father and daughter, mother and son. The latter affords the purest examples of an unalterable tenderness, in no way disturbed by egoistical considerations.

Why do I speak of these things, so banal and so well known? Because there is an unmistakable disposition to deny their significance in life, and to set forth the ideal demanded by society as a fulfilled thing much oftener than it really is fulfilled. But it is preferable for psychology to speak the truth, rather than that this task should be left to the cynic. In any event, this denial refers only to actual life. The arts of narrative and dramatic poetry are still free to make use of the motives that result from a disturbance of this ideal.

It is not to be wondered at that in the case of a large number of people the dream discloses the wish for the removal of the parents, especially the parent of the same sex. We may conclude that it is also present during waking hours, and that it becomes conscious even at times when it is able to mask itself behind another motive, as in the case of the dreamer's sympathy for his father's unnecessary sufferings in example 3. It is seldom that the enmity alone controls the relationship; much more often it recedes behind more tender impulses, by which it is suppressed, and must wait until a dream isolates it. That which the dream shows us in enlarged form as a result of such isolation, shrinks together again after it has been properly docketed in its relation to life as a result of our interpretation (H. Sachs). But we also find this dream wish in places where it has no connection with life, and where the adult, in his waking hours, would never recognize it. The reason for this is that the deepest and most uniform motive for becoming unfriendly, especially between persons of the same sex, has already made its influence felt in earliest childhood.

I mean the love rivalry, with the especial emphasis of the sex character. The son, even as a small child, begins to develop an especial tenderness for his mother, whom he considers as his own property, and feels his father to be a rival who puts into question his individual possession; and in the same manner the little daughter sees in her mother a person who is a disturbing element in her tender relationship with her father, and who occupies a position that she could very well fill herself. One learns from these observations to what early years these ideas extend back— ideas which we designate as the *Oedipus-complex*, because this myth realizes with a very slightly weakened effect the two extreme wishes which grow out of the situation of the son—to kill his father and take his mother to wife. I do not wish to maintain that the Oedipus-complex covers entirely the relation of the child to its parents; this relation can be much more complicated. Furthermore, the Oedipus-complex is more or less well-developed; it may even experience a reversal, but it is a customary and very important factor in the psychic life of the child; and one tends rather to underestimate than to overestimate its influence and the developments which may follow from it. In addition, children frequently react to the Oedipus-idea through stimulation by the parents, who in the placing of their affection are often led by sex-differences, so that the father prefers the daughter, the mother the son; or again, where the marital affection has cooled, and this love is substituted for the outworn love.

One cannot maintain that the world was very grateful to psychoanalytic research for its discovery of the Oedipus-complex. On the contrary, it called forth the strongest resistance on the part of adults; and persons who had neglected to take part in denying this proscribed or tabooed feeling-relationship later made good the omission by taking all value from the complex through false interpretations. According to my unchanged conviction there is nothing to deny and nothing to make more palatable. One should accept the fact, recognized by the Greek myth itself, as inevitable destiny. On the other hand, it is interesting that this Oedipus-complex, cast out of life, was yielded up to poetry and given the freest play. O. Rank has shown in a careful study how this very Oedipus-complex has supplied dramatic literature with a large number of motives in unending variations, derivations and disguises, also in distorted forms such as we recognize to be the work of a censor. We may also ascribe this Oedipus-complex to those dreamers who were so fortunate as to escape in later life these conflicts with their parents, and intimately associated therewith we find what we call the *castration complex*, the reaction to sexual intimidation or restriction, ascribed to the father, of early infantile sexuality.

By applying our former researches to the study of the psychic life of the child, we may expect to find that the origin of other forbidden dream-wishes, of excessive sexual impulses, may be explained in the same manner. Thus we are moved to study the development of sex-life in the child also, and we discover the following from a number of sources: In the first place, it is a mistake to deny that the child has a sexual life, and to take it for granted that sexuality commences with the ripening of the genitals at the time of puberty. On the contrary—the child has from the very beginning a sexual life rich in content and differing in numerous respects from that which is later considered normal. What we call "perverse" in the life of the adult, differs from the normal in the following respects: first, in disregard for the dividing line of species (the gulf between man and animal); second, being insensible to the conventional feeling of disgust; third, the incest-limitation (being prohibited from seeking sexual satisfaction with near blood-relations); fourth, homosexuality, and fifth, transferring the role of the genitals to other organs and other parts of the body. None of these limitations exist in the beginning, but are gradually built up in the course of development and education. The little child is free from them. He knows no unbridgable chasm between man and animal; the arrogance with which man distinguishes himself from the animal is a later acquisition. In the beginning he is not disgusted at the sight of excrement, but slowly learns to be so disgusted under the pressure of education; he lays no special stress on the difference between the sexes, rather accredits to both the same genital formation; he directs his earliest sexual desires and his curiosity toward those persons closest to him, and who are dear to him for various reasons—his parents, brothers and sisters, nurses; and finally, you may observe in him that which later breaks through again, raised now to a love attraction, viz., that he does not expect pleasure from his sexual organs alone, but that many other parts of the body portray the same sensitiveness, are the media of analogous sensations, and are able to play the role of the genitals. The child may, then, be called "polymorphus perverse," and if he makes but slight use of all these impulses, it is, on the one hand, because of their lesser intensity as compared to later life, and on the other hand, because the bringing up of the child immediately and energetically suppresses all his sexual expressions. This suppression continues in theory, so to say, since the grown-ups are careful to control part of the childish sex-expressions, and to disguise another part by misrepresenting its sexual nature until they can deny the whole business. These are often the same persons who discourse violently against all the sexual faults of the child and then at the writing table defend the sexual purity of the same children. Where children are left to themselves or are under the influence of corruption, they often are capable of really conspicuous performances of perverse sexual activity. To be sure, the grown-ups are right in looking upon these things as "childish performances," as "play," for the child is not to be judged as mature and answerable either before the bar of custom or before the law, but these things do exist, they have their significance as indications of innate characteristics as well as causes and furtherances of later developments, they give us an insight into childhood sex-life and thereby into the sex life of man. When we rediscover in the background of our distorted dreams all these perverse wish-impulses, it means only that the dream has in this field traveled back to the infantile condition.

Especially noteworthy among these forbidden wishes are those of incest, i.e., those directed towards sexual intercourse with parents and brothers and sisters. You know what antipathy society feels toward such intercourse, or at least pretends to feel, and what weight is laid on the prohibitions directed against it. The most monstrous efforts have been made to explain this fear of incest. Some have believed that it is due to evolutionary foresight on the part of nature, which is psychically represented by this prohibition, because inbreeding would deteriorate the race-character; others maintained that because of having lived together since early childhood the sexual desire is diverted from the persons under consideration. In both cases, furthermore, the incest-avoidance would be automatically assured, and it would be difficult to understand the need of strict prohibitions, which rather point to the presence of a strong desire. Psychoanalytic research has incontrovertibly shown that the incestuous love choice is rather the first and most customary choice, and that not until later is there any resistance, the source of which probably is to be found in the individual psychology.

Let us sum up what our plunge into child psychology has given us toward the understanding of the dream. We found not only that the materials of forgotten childhood experiences are accessible to the dream, but we saw also that the psychic life of children, with all its peculiarities, its egoism, its incestuous love-choice, etc., continues, for the purposes of the dream, in the unconscious, and that the dream nightly leads us back to this infantile stage. Thus it becomes more certain *that the unconscious in our psychic life is the infantile.* The estranging impression that there is so much evil in man, begins to weaken. This frightful evil is simply the original, primitive, infantile side of psychic life, which we may find in action in children, which we overlook partly because of the slightness of its dimensions, partly because it is lightly considered, since we demand no ethical heights of the child. Since the dream regresses to this stage, it seems to have made apparent the evil that lies in us. But it is only a deceptive appearance by which we have allowed ourselves to be frightened. We are not so evil as we might suspect from the interpretation of dreams.

If the evil impulses of the dream are merely infantilism, a return to the beginnings of our ethical development, since the dream simply makes children of us again in thinking and in feeling, we need not be ashamed of these evil dreams if we are reasonable. But being reasonable is only a part of psychic life. Many things are taking place there that are not reasonable, and so it happens that we are ashamed of such dreams, and unreasonably. We turn them over to the dream-censorship, are ashamed and angry if one of these dreams has in some unusual manner succeeded in penetrating into consciousness in an undistorted form, so that we must recognize it—in fact, we are at times just as ashamed of the distorted dream as we would be if we understood it. Just think of the scandalized opinion of the fine old lady about her uninterpreted dream of "services of love." The problem is not yet solved, and it is still possible that upon further study of the evil in the dream we shall come to some other decision and arrive at another valuation of human nature.

As a result of the whole investigation we grasp two facts, which, however, disclose only the beginnings of new riddles, new doubts. First: the regression of dream-work is not only formal, it is also of greater import. It not only translates our thoughts into a primitive form of expression, but it reawakens the peculiarities of our primitive psychic life, the ancient predominance of the ego, the earliest impulses of our sexual life, even our old intellectual property, if we may consider the symbolic relations as such. And second: We must accredit all these infantilisms which once were governing, and solely governing, to the unconscious, about which our ideas now change and are broadened. Unconscious is no longer a name for what is at that time latent, the unconscious is an especial psychic realm with wish-impulses of its own, with its own method of expression and with a psychic mechanism peculiar to itself, all of which ordinarily are not in force. But the latent dream-thoughts, which we have solved by means of the dream-interpretation, are not of this realm. They are much more nearly the same as any we may have thought in our waking hours. Still they are unconscious; how does one solve this contradiction? We begin to see that a distinction must be made. Something that originates in our conscious life, and that shares its characteristics—we call it the day-remnants—combines in the dream-fabrication with something else out of the realm of the unconscious. Between these two parts the dream-work completes itself. The influencing of the day-remnants by the unconscious necessitates regression. This is the deepest insight into the nature of the dream that we are able to attain without having searched through further psychic realms. The time will soon come, however, when we shall clothe the unconscious character of the latent dream-thought with another name, which shall differentiate it from the unconscious out of the realm of the infantile.

We may, to be sure, propound the question: what forces the psychological activity during sleep to such regression? Why do not the sleep disturbing psychic stimuli do the job without it? And if they must, because of the dream censorship, disguise themselves through old forms of expression which are no longer comprehensible, what is the use of giving new life to old, long-outgrown psychic stimuli, wishes and character types, that is, why the material regression in addition to the formal? The only satisfactory answer would be this, that only in this manner can a dream be built up, that dynamically the dream-stimulus can be satisfied only in this way. But for the time being we have no right to give such an answer.

FOURTEENTH LECTURE

THE DREAM

Wish Fulfillment

MAY I bring to your attention once more the ground we have already covered? How, when we met with dream distortion in the application of our technique, we decided to leave it alone for the time being, and set out to obtain decisive information about the nature of the dream by way of infantile dreams? How, then, armed with the results of this investigation, we attacked dream distortion directly and, I trust, in some measure overcame it? But we must remind ourselves that the results we found along the one way and along the other do not fit together as well as might be. It is now our task to put these two results together and balance them against one another.

From both sources we have seen that the dream-work consists essentially in the transposition of thoughts into an hallucinatory experience. How that can take place is puzzling enough, but it is a problem of general psychology with which we shall not busy ourselves here. We have learned from the dreams of children that the purpose of the dream-work is the satisfaction of one of the sleep-disturbing psychic stimuli by means of a wish fulfillment. We were unable to make a similar statement concerning distorted dreams, until we knew how to interpret them. But from the very beginning we expected to be able to bring the distorted dreams under the same viewpoint as the infantile. The earliest fulfillment of this expectation led us to believe that as a matter of fact all dreams are the dreams of children and that they all work with infantile materials, through childish psychic stimuli and mechanics. Since we consider that we have conquered dream-distortion, we must continue the investigation to see whether our hypothesis of wish-fulfillment holds good for distorted dreams also.

We very recently subjected a number of dreams to interpretation, but left wish-fulfillment entirely out of consideration. I am convinced that the question again and again occurred to you: "What about wish-fulfillment, which ostensibly is the goal of dream-work?" This question is important. It was, in fact, the question of our lay-critics. As you know, humanity has an instinctive antagonism toward intellectual novelties. The expression of such a novelty should immediately be reduced to its narrowest limits, if possible, comprised in a commonplace phrase. Wish-fulfillment has become that phrase for the new dream-science. The layman asks: "Where is the wish-fulfillment?" Immediately, upon having heard that the dream is supposed to be a wish-fulfillment, and indeed, by the very asking of the question, he answers it with a denial. He is at once reminded of countless dream-experiences of his own, where his aversion to the dream was enormous, so that the proposition of psychoanalytic dream-science seems very improbable to him. It is a simple matter to answer the layman that wish-fulfillment cannot be apparent in distorted dreams, but must be sought out, so that it is not recognized until the dream is interpreted. We know, too, that the wishes in these distorted dreams are prohibited wishes, are wishes rejected by the censor and that their existence lit the very cause of the dream distortion and the reason for the intrusion of the dream censor. But it is hard to convince the lay-critic that one may not seek the wish-fulfillment in the dream before the dream has been interpreted. This is continually forgotten. His sceptical attitude toward the theory of wish-fulfillment is really nothing more than a consequence of dream-censorship, a substitute and a result of the denial of this censored dream-wish.

To be sure, even we shall find it necessary to explain to ourselves why there are so many dreams of painful content, and especially dreams of fear. We see here, for the first time, the problem of the affects in the dream, a problem worthy of separate investigation, but which unfortunately cannot be considered here. If the dream is a wish-fulfillment, painful experiences ought to be impossible in the dream; in that the lay-critics apparently are right. But three complications, not thought of by them, must be taken into consideration.

First: It may be that the dream work has not been successful in creating a wish-fulfillment, so that a part of the painful effect of the dream-thought is left over for the manifest dream. Analysis should then show that these thoughts were far more painful even than the dream which was built out of them. This much may be proved in each instance. We admit, then, that the dream work has not achieved its purpose any more than the drink-dream due to the thirst-stimulus has achieved its purpose of satisfying the thirst. One remains thirsty, and must wake up in order to drink. But it was a real dream, it sacrificed nothing of its nature. We must say: "Although strength be lacking, let us praise the will to do." The clearly recognizable intention, at least, remains praiseworthy. Such cases of miscarriage are not unusual. A contributory cause is this, that it is so much more difficult for the dream work to change affect into content in its own sense; the affects often show great resistance, and thus it happens that the dream work has worked the painful content of the dream-thoughts over into a wish-fulfillment, while the painful affect continues in its unaltered form. Hence in dreams of this type the affect does not fit the content at all, and our critics may say the dream is so little a wish-fulfillment that a harmless content may be experienced as painful. In answer to this unintelligible remark we say that the wish-fulfillment tendency in the dream-work appears most prominent, because isolated, in just such dreams. The error is due to the fact that he who does not know neurotics imagines the connection between content and affect as all too intimate, and cannot, therefore, grasp the fact that a content may be altered without any corresponding change in the accompanying affect-expression.

A second, far more important and more extensive consideration, equally disregarded by the layman, is the following: A wish-fulfillment certainly must bring pleasure—but to whom? Naturally, to him who has the wish. But we know from the dreamer that he stands in a very special relationship to his wishes. He casts them aside, censors them, he will have none of them. Their fulfillment gives him no pleasure, but only the opposite. Experience then shows that this opposite, which must still be explained, appears in the form of fear. The dreamer in his relation to his dream-wishes can be compared only to a combination of two persons bound together by some strong common quality. Instead of further explanations I shall give you a well-known fairy tale, in which you will again find the relationships I have mentioned. A good fairy promises a poor couple, husband and wife, to fulfill their first three wishes. They are overjoyed, and determine to choose their three wishes with great care. But the woman allows herself to be led astray by the odor of cooking sausages emanating from the next cottage, and wishes she had a couple of such sausages. Presto! they are there. This is the first wish-fulfillment. Now the husband becomes angry, and in his bitterness wishes that the sausages might hang from the end of her nose. This, too, is accomplished, and the sausages cannot be removed from their new location. So this is the second wish-fulfillment, but the wish is that of the husband. The wife is very uncomfortable because of the fulfillment of this wish. You know how the fairy tale continues. Since both husband and wife are fundamentally one, the third wish must be that the sausages be removed from the nose of the wife. We could make use of this fairy tale any number of times in various connections; here it serves only as an illustration of the possibility that the wish-fulfillment for the one personality may lead to an aversion on the part of the other, if the two do not agree with one another.

It will not be difficult now to come to a better understanding of the anxiety-dream. We shall make one more observation, then we shall come to a conclusion to which many things lead. The observation is that the anxiety dreams often have a content which is entirely free from distortion and in which the censorship is, so to speak, eluded. The anxiety dream is ofttimes an undisguised wish-fulfillment, not, to be sure, of an accepted, but of a discarded wish. The anxiety development has stepped into the place of the censorship. While one may assert of the infantile dream that it is the obvious fulfillment of a wish that has gained admittance, and of the distorted dream that it is the disguised fulfillment of a suppressed wish, he must say of the anxiety dream that the only suitable formula is this, that it is the obvious fulfillment of a suppressed wish. Anxiety is the mark which shows that the suppressed wish showed itself stronger than the censorship, that it put through its wish-fulfillment despite the censorship, or was about to put it through. We understand that what is wish-fulfillment for the suppressed wish is for us, who are on the side of the dream-censor, only a painful sensation and a cause for antagonism. The anxiety which occurs in dreams is, if you wish, anxiety because of the strength of these otherwise suppressed wishes. Why this antagonism arises in the form of anxiety cannot be discovered from a study of the dream alone; one must obviously study anxiety from other sources.

What holds true for the undistorted anxiety dream we may assume to be true also of those dreams which have undergone partial distortion, and of the other dreams of aversion whose painful impressions very probably denote approximations of anxiety. The anxiety dream is usually also a dream that causes waking; we habitually interrupt sleep before the suppressed wish of the dream has accomplished its entire fulfillment in opposition to the censorship. In this case the execution of the dream is unsuccessful, but this does not change its nature. We have likened the dream to the night watchman or sleep-defender who wishes to protect our sleep from being disturbed. The night watchman, too, sometimes wakes the sleeper when he feels himself too weak to drive away the disturbance or danger all by himself. Yet we are often able to remain asleep, even when the dream begins to become suspicious, and begins to assume the form of anxiety. We say to ourselves in our sleep: "It's only a dream," and we sleep on.

When does it happen that the dream-wish is in a position to overpower this censorship? The conditions for this may be just as easily furnished by the dream-wish as by the dream-censorship. The wish may, for unknown reasons, become irresistible; but one gets the impression that more frequently the attitude of the dream censorship is to blame for this disarrangement in the relations of the forces. We have already heard that the censorship works with varying intensity in each single instance, that it handles each element with a different degree of strictness; now we should like to add the proposition that it is an extremely variable thing and does not exert equal force on every occasion against the same objectionable element. If on occasion the censorship feels itself powerless with respect to a dream-wish which threatens to over-ride it, then, instead of distortion, it makes use of the final means at its disposal, it destroys the sleep condition by the development of anxiety.

And now it occurs to us that we know absolutely nothing yet as to why these evil, depraved wishes are aroused just at night, in order that they may disturb our sleep. The answer can only be an assumption which is based on the nature of the condition of sleep. During the day the heavy pressure of a censorship weighs upon these wishes, making it impossible, as a rule, for them to express themselves in any manner. At night, evidently, this censorship is withdrawn for the benefit of the single sleep-wish, in the same manner as are all the other interests of psychic life, or at least placed in a position of very minor importance. The forbidden wishes must thank this noctural deposition of the censor for being able to raise their heads again. There are nervous persons troubled with insomnia who admit that their sleeplessness was in the beginning voluntary. They did not trust themselves to fall asleep, because they were afraid of their dreams, that is, of the results due to a slackening of the censorship. So you can readily see that this withdrawal of the censor does not in itself signify rank carelessness. Sleep weakens our power to move; our evil intentions, even if they do begin to stir, can accomplish nothing but a dream, which for practical purposes is harmless, and the highly sensible remark of the sleepers, a night-time remark indeed, but not a part of the dream life, "it is only a dream," is reminiscent of this quieting circumstance. So let us grant this, and sleep on.

If, thirdly, you recall the concept that the dreamer, struggling against his wishes, is to be compared to a summation of two separate persons, in some manner closely connected, you will be able to grasp the further possibility of how a thing which is highly unpleasant, namely, punishment, may be accomplished by wish-fulfillment. Here again the fairy tale of the three wishes can be of service to us: the sausages on the plate are the direct wish-fulfillment of the first person, the woman; the sausages at the end of her nose are the wish-fulfillment of the second person, the husband, but at the same time the punishment for the stupid wish of the woman. Among the neurotics we find again the motivation of the third wish, which remains in fairy tales only. There are many such punishment-tendencies in the psychic life of man; they are very powerful, and we may make them responsible for some of our painful dreams. Perhaps you now say that at this rate, not very much of the famed wish-fulfillment is left. But upon closer view you will admit that you are wrong. In contrast to the many-sided to be discussed, of what the dream might be—and, according to numerous authors, is—the solution (wish-fulfillment, anxiety-fulfillment, punishment-fulfillment) is indeed very restricted. That is why anxiety is the direct antithesis of the wish, why antitheses are so closely allied in association and why they occur together in the unconscious, as we have heard; and that is why punishment, too, is a wish-fulfillment of the other, the censoring person.

On the whole, then, I have made no concessions to your protestation against the theory of wish-fulfillment. We are bound, however, to establish wish-fulfillment in every dream no matter how distorted, and we certainly do not wish to withdraw from this task. Let us go back to the dream, already interpreted, of the three bad theatre tickets for 1 Fl. 50 Kr. from which we have already learned so much. I hope you still remember it. A lady who tells her husband during the day that her friend Elise, only three months younger than herself, has become engaged, dreams she is in the theatre with her husband. Half the parquet is empty. Her husband says, "Elise and her fiancé wanted to go to the theatre, too, but couldn't because they could get only poor seats, three for one gulden and a half." She was of the opinion that that wasn't so unfortunate. We discovered that the dream-thought originated in her discontent at having married too soon, and the fact that she was dissatisfied with her husband. We may be curious as to the manner in which these thoughts have been worked over into a wish-fulfillment, and where their traces may be found in the manifest content. Now we know that the element "too soon, premature" is eliminated from the dream by the censor. The empty parquet is a reference to it. The puzzling "three for 1 Fl. 50 Kr." is now, with the help of symbolism which we have since learned, more understandable.[36] The "3" really means a husband, and the manifest element is easy to translate: to buy a husband for her dowry ("I could have bought one ten times better for my dowry"). The marriage is obviously replaced by going into the theatre. "Buying the tickets too soon" directly takes the place of the premature marriage. This substitution is the work of the wish-fulfillment. Our dreamer was not always so dissatisfied with her early marriage as she was on the day she received news of the engagement of her friend. At the time she was proud of her marriage and felt herself more favored than her friend. Naive girls have frequently confided to their friends after their engagement that soon they, too, will be able to go to all the plays hitherto forbidden, and see everything. The desire to see plays, the curiosity that makes its appearance here, was certainly in the beginning directed towards sex matters, the sex-life, especially the sex-life of the parents, and then became a strong motive which impelled the girl to an early marriage. In this way the visit to the theatre becomes an obvious representative substitute for being married. In the momentary annoyance at her early marriage she recalls the time when the early marriage was a wish-fulfillment for her, because she had satisfied her curiosity; and she now replaces the marriage, guided by the old wish-impulse, with the going to the theatre.

We may say that we have not sought out the simplest example as proof of a hidden wish-fulfillment. We would have to proceed in analogous manner with other distorted dreams. I cannot do that for you, and simply wish to express the conviction that it will be successful everywhere. But I wish to continue along this theoretical line. Experience has taught me that it is one of the most dangerous phases of the entire dream science, and that many contradictions and misunderstandings are connected therewith. Besides, you are perhaps still under the impression that I have retracted a part of my declaration, in that I said that the dream is a fulfilled wish or its opposite, an actualized anxiety or punishment, and you will think this is the opportunity to compel further reservations of me. I have also heard complaints that I am too abrupt about things which appear evident to me, and that for that reason I do not present the thing convincingly enough.

If a person has gone thus far with us in dream-interpretation, and accepted everything that has been offered, it is not unusual for him to call a halt at wish-fulfillment, and say, "Granted that in every instance the dream has a meaning, and that this meaning can be disclosed by psychoanalytic technique, why must this dream, despite all evidence to the contrary, always be forced into the formula of wish-fulfillment? Why might not the meaning of this nocturnal thought be as many-sided as thought is by day; why may not the dream in one case express a fulfilled wish, in another, as you yourself say, the opposite thereof, an actualized anxiety; or why may it not correspond to a resolution, a warning, a reflection with its pro's and con's, a reproach, a goad to conscience, an attempt to prepare oneself for a contemplated performance, etc? Why always nothing more than a wish, or at best, its opposite?"

One might maintain that a difference of opinion on these points is of no great importance, so long as we are at one otherwise. We might say that it is enough to have discovered the meaning of the dream, and the way to recognize it; that it is a matter of no importance, if we have too narrowly limited this meaning. But this is not so. A misunderstanding of this point strikes at the nature of our knowledge of the dream, and endangers its worth for the understanding of neuroses. Then, too, that method of approach which is esteemed in the business world as genteel is out of place in scientific endeavors, and harmful.

My first answer to the question why the dream may not be many-sided in its meaning is the usual one in such instances: I do not know why it should not be so. I would not be opposed to such a state of affairs. As far as I am concerned, it could well be true. Only one small matter prevents this broader and more comfortable explanation of the dream—namely, that as a matter of fact it isn't so. My second answer emphasizes the fact that the assumption that the dream corresponds to numerous forms of thought and intellectual operations is no stranger to me. In a story about a sick person I once reported a dream that occurred three nights running and then stopped, and I explained this suppression by saying that the dream corresponded to a resolution which had no reason to recur after having been carried out. More recently I published a dream which corresponded to a confession. How is it possible for me to contradict myself, and maintain that the dream is always only a fulfilled wish?

I do that, because I do not wish to admit a stupid misunderstanding which might cost us the fruits of all our labors with regard to the dream, a misunderstanding which confuses the dream with the latent dream-thought and affirms of the dream something that applies specifically and solely to the latter. For it is entirely correct that the dream can represent, and be replaced by all those things we enumerated: a resolution, a warning, reflection, preparation, an attempt to solve a problem, etc. But if you look closely, you will recognize that all these things are true only of the latent dream thoughts, which have been changed about in the dream. You learn from the interpretation of the dreams that the person's unconscious thinking is occupied with such resolutions, preparations, reflections, etc., out of which the dream-work then builds the dream. If you are not at the time interested in the dream-work, but are very much interested in the unconscious thought-work of man, you eliminate the dream-work, and say of the dream, for all practical purposes quite correctly, that it corresponds to a warning, a resolution, etc. This often happens in psychoanalytic activity. People endeavor for the most part only to destroy the dream form, and to substitute in its place in the sequence the latent thoughts out of which the dream was made.

Thus we learn, from the appreciation of the latent dream-thoughts, that all the highly complicated psychic acts we have enumerated can go on unconsciously, a result as wonderful as it is confusing.

But to return, you are right only if you admit that you have made use of an abbreviated form of speech, and if you do not believe that you must connect the many-sidedness we have mentioned with the essence of the dream. When you speak of the dream you must mean either the manifest dream, i.e., the product of the dream-work, or at most the dream-work itself—that psychic occurrence which forms the manifest dream out of the latent dream thought. Any other use of the word is a confusion of concept that can only cause trouble. If your assertions refer to the latent thoughts back of the dream, say so, and do not cloud the problem of the dream by using such a faulty means of expression. The latent dream thoughts are the material which the dream-work remolds into the manifest dream. Why do you insist upon confusing the material with the work that makes use of it? Are you any better off than those who knew only the product of this work, and could explain neither where it came from nor how it was produced?

The only essential thing in the dream is the dream-work that has had its influence upon the thought-material. We have no right to disregard it theoretically even if, in certain practical situations, we may fail to take it into account. Analytic observation, too, shows that the dream-work never limits itself to translating these thoughts in the archaic or regressive mode of expression known to you. Rather it regularly adds something which does not belong to the latent thoughts of waking, but which is the essential motive of dream-formation. This indispensable ingredient is at the same time the unconscious wish, for the fulfillment of which the dream content is rebuilt. The dream may be any conceivable thing, if you take into account only the thoughts represented by it, warning, resolution, preparation, etc.; it is also always the fulfillment of an unknown wish, and it is this only if you look upon it as the result of the dream-work. A dream is never itself a resolution, a warning, and no more—but always a resolution, etc., translated into an archaic form of expression with the help of the unconscious wish, and changed about for the purpose of fulfilling this wish. The one characteristic, wish-fulfillment, is constant; the other may vary; it may itself be a wish at times, so that the dream, with the aid of an unconscious wish, presents as fulfilled a latent wish out of waking hours.

I understand all this very well, but I do not know whether or not I shall be successful in making you understand it as well. I have difficulties, too, in proving it to you. This cannot be done without, on the one hand, careful analysis of many dreams, and on the other hand this most difficult and most important point of our conception of the dream cannot be set forth convincingly without reference to things to follow. Can you, in fact, believe that taking into consideration the intimate relationship of all things, one is able to penetrate deeply into the nature of one thing without having carefully considered other things of a very similar nature? Since we know nothing as yet about the closest relatives of the dream, neurotic symptoms, we must once again content ourselves with what has already been accomplished. I want to explain one more example to you, and propose a new viewpoint.

Let us again take up that dream to which we have several times recurred, the dream of the three theatre tickets for 1 Fl. 50 Kr. I can assure you that I took this example quite unpremeditatedly at first. You are acquainted with the latent dream thoughts: annoyance, upon hearing that her friend had just now become engaged, at the thought that she herself had hurried so to be married; contempt for her husband; the idea that she might have had a better one had she waited. We also know the wish, which made a dream out of these thoughts—it is "curiosity to see," being permitted to go to the theatre, very likely a derivation from the old curiosity finally to know just what happens when one is married. This curiosity, as is well known, regularly directs itself in the case of children to the sex-life of the parents. It is an impulse of childhood, and in so far as it persists later, an impulse whose roots reach back into the infantile. But that day's news played no part in awaking the curiosity, it awoke only annoyance and regret. This wish impulse did not have anything to do immediately with the latent dream thoughts, and we could fit the result of the dream interpretation into the analysis without considering the wish impulse at all. But then, the annoyance itself was not capable of producing the dream; a dream could not be derived from the thought: "It was stupid to marry so soon," except by reviving the old wish finally to see what happens when one is married. The wish then formed the dream content, in that it replaced marriage by going to the theatre, and gave it the form of an earlier wish-fulfillment: "so now I may go to the theatre and see all the forbidden things, and you may not. I am married and you must wait." In such a manner the present situation was transposed into its opposite, an old triumph put into the place of the recent defeat. Added thereto was a satisfied curiosity amalgamated with a satisfied egoistic sense of rivalry. This satisfaction determines the manifest dream content in which she really is sitting in the theatre, and her friend was unable to get tickets. Those bits of dream content are affixed to this satisfaction situation as unfitting and inexplicable modifications, behind which the latent dream thoughts still hide. Dream interpretation must take into consideration everything that serves toward the representation of the wish-fulfillment and must reconstruct from these suggestions the painful latent dream-thought.

The observation I now wish to make is for the purpose of drawing your attention to the latent, dream thoughts, now pushed to the fore. I beg of you not to forget first, that the dreamer is unconscious of them, second, they are entirely logical and continuous, so that they may be understood as a comprehensible reaction to the dream occasion, third, that they may have the value of any desired psychic impulse or intellectual operation. I shall now designate these thoughts more forcibly than before as "day-remnants"; the dreamer may acknowledge them or not. I now separate day-remnants and latent dream thoughts in accordance with our previous usage of calling everything that we discover in interpreting the dream "latent dream thoughts," while the day-remnants are only a part of the latent dream thoughts. Then our conception goes to show that something additional has been added to the day-remnants, something which also belonged to the unconscious, a strong but suppressed wish impulse, and it is this alone that has made possible the dream fabrication. The influence of this wish impulse on the day-remnants creates the further participation of the latent dream thoughts, thoughts which no longer appear rational and understandable in relation to waking life.

In explaining the relationship of the day-remnants to the unconscious wish I have made use of a comparison which I can only repeat here. Every undertaking requires a capitalist, who defrays the expenses, and an entrepreneur, who has the idea and understands how to carry it out. The role of the capitalist in the dream fabrication is always played by the unconscious wish; it dispenses the psychic energy for dream-building. The actual worker is the day-remnant, which determines how the expenditure is to be made. Now the capitalist may himself have the idea and the particularized knowledge, or the entrepreneur may have the capital. This simplifies the practical situation, but makes its theoretical comprehension more difficult. In economics we always distinguish between the capitalist and the entrepreneur aspect in a single person, and thus we reconstruct the fundamental situation which was the point of departure for our comparison. In dream-fabrication the same variations occur. I shall leave their further development to you.

We can go no further here, for you have probably long been disturbed by a reflection which deserves to be heard. Are the day-remnants, you ask, really unconscious in the same sense as the unconscious wish which is essential to making them suitable for the dream? You discern correctly. Here lies the salient point of the whole affair. They are not unconscious in the same sense. The dream wish belongs to a different unconsciousness, that which we have recognized as of infantile origin, fitted out with special mechanisms. It is entirely appropriate to separate these two types of unconsciousness and give them different designations. But let us rather wait until we have become acquainted with the field of neurotic symptoms. If people say one unconsciousness is fantastic, what will they say when we acknowledge that we arrived at our conclusions by using two kinds of unconsciousness?

Let us stop here. Once more you have heard something incomplete; but is there not hope in the thought that this science has a continuation which will be brought to light either by ourselves or by those to follow? And have not we ourselves discovered a sufficient number of new and surprising things?

FIFTEENTH LECTURE

THE DREAM

Doubtful Points and Criticism

LET us not leave the subject of dreams before we have touched upon the most common doubts and uncertainties which have arisen in connection with the new ideas and conceptions we have discussed up to this point. The more attentive members of the audience probably have already accumulated some material bearing upon this.

1. You may have received the impression that the results of our work of interpretation of the dream have left so much that is uncertain, despite our close adherence to technique, that a true translation of the manifest dream into the latent dream thoughts is thereby rendered impossible. In support of this you will point out that in the first place, one never knows whether a specific element of the dream is to be taken literally or symbolically, since those elements which are used symbolically do not, because of that fact, cease to be themselves. But if one has no objective standard by which to decide this, the interpretation is, as to this point, left to the discretion of the dream interpreter. Moreover, because of the way in which the dream work combines opposites, it is always uncertain whether a specific dream element is to be taken in the positive or the negative sense, whether it is to be understood as itself or as its opposite. Hence this is another opportunity for the exercise of the interpreter's discretion. In the third place, in consequence of the frequency with which every sort of inversion is practised in the dream, the dream interpreter is at liberty to assume such an inversion at any point of the dream he pleases. And finally you will say, you have heard that one is seldom sure that the interpretation which is found is the only possible one. There is danger of overlooking a thoroughly admissible second interpretation of the same dream. Under these circumstances, you will conclude there is a scope left for the discretion of the interpreter, the breadth of which seems incompatible with the objective accuracy of the results. Or you may also conclude that the fault does not rest with the dream but that the inadequacies of our dream interpretation result from errors in our conceptions and hypotheses.

All your material is irreproachable, but I do not believe that it justifies your conclusions in two directions, namely, that dream interpretation as we practice it is sacrificed to arbitrariness and that the deficiency of our results makes the justification of our method doubtful. If you will substitute for the arbitrariness of the interpreter, his skill, his experience, his comprehension, I agree with you. We shall surely not be able to dispense with some such personal factor, particularly not in difficult tasks of dream interpretation. But this same state of affairs exists also in other scientific occupations. There is no way in which to make sure that one man will not wield a technique less well, or utilize it more fully, than another. What might, for example, impress you as arbitrariness in the interpretation of symbols, is compensated for by the fact that as a rule the connection of the dream thoughts among themselves, the connection of the dream with the life of the dreamer, and the whole psychic situation in which the dream occurs, chooses just one of the possible interpretations advanced and rejects the others as useless for its purposes. The conclusion drawn from the inadequacies of dream interpretation, that our hypotheses are wrong, is weakened by an observation which shows that the ambiguity and indefiniteness of the dream is rather characteristic and necessarily to be expected.

Recollect that we said that the dream work translates the dream thoughts into primitive expressions analogous to picture writing. All these primitive systems of expression are, however, subject to such indefiniteness and ambiguities, but it does not follow that we are justified in doubting their usefulness. You know that the fusion of opposites by the dream-work is analogous to the so-called "antithetical meaning of primitive words," in the oldest languages. The philologist, R. Abel (1884), whom we have to thank for this point of view, admonishes us not to believe that the meaning of the communication which one person made to another when using such ambiguous words was necessarily unclear. Tone and gesture used in connection with the words would have left no room for doubt as to which of the two opposites the speaker intended to communicate. In writing, where gesture is lacking, it was replaced by a supplementary picture sign not intended to be spoken, as for example by the picture of a little man squatting lazily or standing erect, according to whether the ambiguous hieroglyphic was to mean "weak" or "strong." It was in this way that one avoided any misunderstanding despite the ambiguity of the sounds and signs.

We recognize in the ancient systems of expression, e.g., the writings of those oldest languages, a number of uncertainties which we would not tolerate in our present-day writings. Thus in many Semitic writings only the consonants of words are indicated. The reader had to supply the omitted vowels according to his knowledge and the context. Hieroglyphic writing does not proceed in exactly this way, but quite similarly, and that is why the pronunciation of old Egyptian has remained unknown to us. The holy writings of the Egyptians contain still other uncertainties. For example, it is left to the discretion of the writer whether or not he shall arrange the pictures from right to left or from left to right. To be able to read we have to follow the rule that we must depend upon the faces of the figures, birds, and the like. The writer, however, could also arrange the picture signs in vertical rows, and in inscriptions on small objects he was guided by considerations of beauty and proportion further to change the order of the signs. Probably the most confusing feature of hieroglyphic writing is to be found in the fact that there is no space between words. The pictures stretch over the page at uniform distances from one another, and generally one does not know whether a sign belongs to what has gone before or is the beginning of a new word. Persian cuneiform writing, on the other hand, makes use of an oblique wedge sign to separate the words.

The Chinese tongue and script is exceedingly old, but still used by four hundred million people. Please do not think I understand anything about it. I have only informed myself concerning it because I hoped to find analogies to the indefinite aspects of the dream. Nor was I disappointed. The Chinese language is filled with so many vagaries that it strikes terror into our hearts. It consists, as is well known, of a number of syllable sounds which are spoken singly or are combined in twos. One of the chief dialects has about four hundred such sounds. Now since the vocabulary of this dialect is estimated at about four thousand words, it follows that every sound has on an average of ten different meanings, some less but others, consequently, more. Hence there are a great number of ways of avoiding a multiplicity of meaning, since one cannot guess from the context alone which of the ten meanings of the syllable sound the speaker intended to convey to the hearer. Among them are the combining of two sounds into a compounded word and the use of four different "tones" with which to utter these syllables. For our purposes of comparison, it is still more interesting to note that this language has practically no grammar. It is impossible to say of a one-syllable word whether it is a noun, a verb, or an adjective, and we find none of those changes in the forms of the words by means of which we might recognize sex, number, ending, tense or mood. The language, therefore, might be said to consist of raw material, much in the same manner as our thought language is broken up by the dream work into its raw materials when the expressions of relationship are left out. In the Chinese, in all cases of vagueness the decision is left to the understanding of the hearer, who is guided by the context. I have secured an example of a Chinese saying which, literally translated, reads: "Little to be seen, much to wonder at." That is not difficult to understand. It may mean, "The less a man has seen, the more he finds to wonder at," or, "There is much to admire for the man who has seen little." Naturally, there is no need to choose between these two translations, which differ only in grammar. Despite these uncertainties, we are assured, the Chinese language is an extraordinarily excellent medium for the expression of thought. Vagueness does not, therefore, necessarily lead to ambiguity.

Now we must certainly admit that the condition of affairs is far less favorable in the expression-system of the dream than in these ancient languages and writings. For, after all, these latter are really designed for communication, that is to say, they were always intended to be understood, no matter in what way and with what aids. But it is just this characteristic which the dream lacks. The dream does not want to tell anyone anything, it is no vehicle of communication, it is, on the contrary, constructed so as not to be understood. For that reason we must not be surprised or misled if we should discover that a number of the ambiguities and vagaries of the dream do not permit of determination. As the one specific gain of our comparison, we have only the realization that such uncertainties as people tried to make use of in objecting to the validity of our dream interpretation, are rather the invariable characteristic of all primitive systems of expression.

How far the dream can really be understood can be determined only by practice and experience. My opinion is, that that is very far indeed, and the comparison of results which correctly trained analysts have gathered confirms my view. The lay public, even that part of the lay public which is interested in science, likes, in the face of the difficulties and uncertainties of a scientific task, to make what I consider an unjust show of its superior scepticism. Perhaps not all of you are acquainted with the fact that a similar situation arose in the history of the deciphering of the Babylonian-Assyrian inscriptions. There was a period then when public opinion went far in declaring the decipherors of cuneiform writing to be visionaries and the whole research a "fraud." But in the year 1857 the Royal Asiatic Society made a decisive test. It challenged the four most distinguished decipherors of cuneiform writing, Rawlinson, Hincks, Fox Talbot and Oppert, each to send to it in a sealed envelope his independent translation of a newly discovered inscription, and the Society was then able to testify, after having made a comparison of the four readings, that their agreement was sufficiently marked to justify confidence in what already had been accomplished, and faith in further progress. At this the mockery of the learned lay world gradually came to an end and the confidence in the reading of cuneiform documents has grown appreciably since then.

2. A second series of objections is firmly grounded in the impression from which you too probably are not free, that a number of the solutions of dream interpretations which we find it necessary to make seem forced, artificial, far-fetched, in other words, violent or even comical or jocose. These comments are so frequent that I shall choose at random the latest example which has come to my attention. Recently, in free Switzerland, the director of a boarding-school was relieved of his position on account of his active interest in psychoanalysis. He raised objections and a Berne newspaper made public the judgment of the school authorities. I quote from that article some sentences which apply to psychoanalysis: "Moreover, we are surprised at the many far-fetched and artificial examples as found in the aforementioned book of Dr. Pfister of Zurich.... Thus, it certainly is a cause of surprise when the director of a boarding-school so uncritically accepts all these assertions and apparent proofs." These observations are offered as the decisions of "one who judges calmly." I rather think this calm is "artificial." Let us examine these remarks more closely in the hope that a little reflection and knowledge of the subject can be no detriment to calm judgment.

It is positively refreshing to see how quickly and unerringly some individuals can judge a delicate question of abstruse psychology by first impressions. The interpretations seem to them far-fetched and forced, they do not please them, so the interpretations are wrong and the whole business of interpretation amounts to nothing. No fleeting thought ever brushes the other possibility, that these interpretations must appear as they are for good reasons, which would give rise to the further question of what these good reasons might be.

The content thus judged generally relates to the results of displacement, with which you have become acquainted as the strongest device of the dream censor. It is with the help of displacements that the dream censor creates substitute-formations which we have designated as allusions. But they are allusions which are not easily recognized as such, and from which it is not easy to find one's way back to the original and which are connected with this original by means of the strangest, most unusual, most superficial associations. In all of these cases, however, it is a question of matters which are to be hidden, which were intended for concealment; this is what the dream censor aims to do. We must not expect to find a thing that has been concealed in its accustomed place in the spot where it belongs. In this respect the Commissions for the Surveillance of Frontiers now in office are more cunning than the Swiss school authorities. In their search for documents and maps they are not content to search through portfolios and letter cases but they also take into account the possibility that spies and smugglers might carry such severely proscribed articles in the most concealed parts of their clothing, where they certainly do not belong, as for example between the double soles of their boots. If the concealed objects are found in such a place, they certainly are very far-fetched, but nevertheless they have been "fetched."

If we recognize that the most remote, the most extraordinary associations between the latent dream element and its manifest substitute are possible, associations appearing ofttimes comical, ofttimes witty, we follow in so doing a wealth of experience derived from examples whose solutions we have, as a rule, not found ourselves. Often it is not possible to give such interpretations from our own examples. No sane person could guess the requisite association. The dreamer either gives us the translation with one stroke by means of his immediate association—he can do this, for this substitute formation was created by his mind—or he provides us with so much material that the solution no longer demands any special astuteness but forces itself upon us as inevitable. If the dreamer does not help us in either of these two ways, then indeed the manifest element in question remains forever incomprehensible to us. Allow me to give you one more such example of recent occurrence. One of my patients lost her father during the time that she was undergoing treatment. Since then she has made use of every opportunity to bring him back to life in her dreams. In one of her dreams her father appears in a certain connection, of no further importance here, and says, "*It is a quarter past eleven, it is half past eleven, it is quarter of twelve.*" All she can think of in connection with this curious incident is the recollection that her father liked to see his grown-up children appear punctually at the general meal hour. That very thing probably had some connection with the dream element, but permitted of no conclusion as to its source. Judging from the situation of the treatment at that time, there was a justified suspicion that a carefully suppressed critical rebellion against her loved and respected father played its part in this dream. Continuing her associations, and apparently far afield from topics relevant to the dream, the dreamer relates that yesterday many things of a psychological nature had been discussed in her presence, and that a relative made the remark: "The cave man (*Urmensch*) continues to live in all of us." Now we think we understand. That gave her an excellent opportunity of picturing her father as continuing to live. So in the dream she made of him a clockman (*Uhrmensch*) by having him announce the quarter-hours at noon time.

You may not be able to disregard the similarity which this examples bears to a pun, and it really has happened frequently that the dreamer's pun is attributed to the interpreter. There are still other examples in which it is not at all easy to decide whether one is dealing with a joke or a dream. But you will recall that the same doubt confronted us when we were dealing with slips of the tongue. A man tells us a dream of his, that his uncle, while they were sitting in the latter's *auto*mobile, gave him a kiss. He very quickly supplies the interpretation himself. It means "*auto*-eroticism," (a term taken from the study of the libido, or love impulse, and designating satisfaction of that impulse without an external object). Did this man permit himself to make fun of us and give out as a dream a pun that occurred to him? I do not believe so; he really dreamed it. Whence comes the astounding similarity? This question at one time led me quite a ways from my path, by making it necessary for me to make a thorough investigation of the problem of humor itself. By so doing I came to the conclusion that the origin of wit lies in a foreconscious train of thought which is left for a moment to unconscious manipulation, from which it then emerges as a joke. Under the influence of the unconscious it experiences the workings of the mechanisms there in force, namely, of condensation and displacement, that is, of the same processes which we found active in the dream work, and it is to this agreement that we are to ascribe the similarity between wit and the dream, wherever it occurs. The unintentional "dream joke" has, however, none of the pleasure-giving quality of the ordinary joke. Why that is so, greater penetration into the study of wit may teach you. The "dream joke" seems a poor joke to us, it does not make us laugh, it leaves us cold.

Here we are also following in the footsteps of ancient dream interpretation, which has left us, in addition to much that is useless, many a good example of dream interpretation we ourselves cannot surpass. I am now going to tell you a dream of historical importance which Plutarch and Artemidorus of Daldis both tell concerning Alexander the Great, with certain variations. When the King was engaged in besieging the city of Tyre (322 B.C.), which was being stubbornly defended, he once dreamed that he saw a dancing satyr. Aristandros, his dream interpreter, who accompanied the army, interpreted this dream for him by making of the word *Satyros*, σά Τύρος, "Thine is Tyre," and thus promising him a triumph over the city. Alexander allowed himself to be influenced by this interpretation to continue the siege, and finally captured Tyre. The interpretation, which seems artificial enough, was without doubt the correct one.

3. I can imagine that it will make a special impression on you to hear that objections to our conception of the dream have been raised also by persons who, as psychoanalysts, have themselves been interested in the interpretation of dreams. It would have been too extraordinary if so pregnant an opportunity for new errors had remained unutilized, and thus, owing to comprehensible confusions and unjustified generalizations, there have been assertions made which, in point of incorrectness are not far behind the medical conception of dreams. One of these you already know. It is the declaration that the dream is occupied with the dreamer's attempts at adaptation to his present environment, and attempts to solve future problems, in

other words, that the dream follows a "prospective tendency" (A. Maeder). We have already shown that this assertion is based upon a confusion of the dream with the latent thoughts of the dream, that as a premise it overlooks the existence of the dream-work. In characterizing that psychic activity which is unconscious and to which the latent thoughts of the dream belong, the above assertion is no novelty, nor is it exhaustive, for this unconscious psychic activity occupies itself with many other things besides preparation for the future. A much worse confusion seems to underlie the assurance that back of every dream one finds the "death-clause," or death-wish. I am not quite certain what this formula is meant to indicate, but I suppose that back of it is a confusion of the dream with the whole personality of the dreamer.

An unjustified generalization, based on few good examples, is the pronouncement that every dream permits of two interpretations, one such as we have explained, the so-called psychoanalytic, and another, the so-called anagogical or mystical, which ignores the instinctive impulses and aims at a representation of the higher psychic functions (V. Silberer). There are such dreams, but you will try in vain to extend this conception to even a majority of the dreams. But after everything you have heard, the statement will seem very incomprehensible that all dreams can be interpreted bisexually, that is, as the concurrence of two tendencies which may be designated as male and female (A. Adler). To be sure, there are a few such dreams, and you may learn later that these are built up in the manner of certain hysterical symptoms. I mention all these newly discovered general characteristics of the dream in order to warn you against them or at least in order not to leave you in doubt as to how I judge them.

4. At one time the objective value of dream research was called into question by the observation that patients undergoing analysis accommodate the content of their dreams to the favorite theories of their physicians, so that some dream predominantly of sexual impulses, others of the desire for power and still others even of rebirth (W. Stekel). The weight of this observation is diminished by the consideration that people dreamed before there was such a thing as a psychoanalytic treatment to influence their dreams, and that those who are now undergoing treatment were also in the habit of dreaming before the treatment was commenced. The meaning of this novel discovery can soon be recognized as a matter of course and as of no consequence for the theory of the dream. Those day-remnants which give rise to the dream are the overflow from the strong interest of the waking life. If the remarks of the physician and the stimuli which he gives have become significant to the patient under analysis, then they become a part of the day's remnants, can serve as psychic stimuli for the formation of a dream along with other, emotionally-charged, unsolved interests of the day, and operate much as do the somatic stimuli which act upon the sleeper during his sleep. Just like these other incitors of the dream, the sequence of ideas which the physician sets in motion may appear in the manifest content, or may be traced in the latent content of the dream. Indeed, we know that one can produce dreams experimentally, or to speak more accurately, one can insert into the dream a part of the dream material.

Thus the analyst in influencing his patients, merely plays the role of an experimenter in the manner of Mourly Vold, who places the limbs of his subjects in certain positions.

One can often influence the dreamer as to the *subject-matter* of his dream, but one can never influence *what he will dream* about it. The mechanism of the dream-work and the unconscious wish that is hidden in the dream are beyond the reach of all foreign influences. We already realized, when we evaluated the dreams caused by bodily stimuli, that the peculiarity and self-sufficiency of the dream life shows itself in the reaction with which the dream retorts to the bodily or physical stimuli which are presented. The statement here discussed, which aims to throw doubt upon the objectivity of dream research, is again based on a confusion—this time of the whole dream with the dream material.

This much, ladies and gentlemen, I wanted to tell you concerning the problems of the dream. You will suspect that I have omitted a great deal, and have yourselves discovered that I had to be inconclusive on almost all points. But that is due to the relation which the phenomena of the dream have to those of the neuroses. We studied the dream by way of introduction to the study of the neuroses, and that was surely more correct than the reverse would have been. But just as the dream prepares us for the understanding of the neuroses, so in turn the correct evaluation of the dream can only be gained after a knowledge of neurotic phenomena has been won.

I do not know what you will think about this, but I must assure you that I do not regret having taken so much of your interest and of your available time for the problems of the dream. There is no other field in which one can so quickly become convinced of the correctness of the assertions by which psychoanalysis stands or falls. It will take the strenuous labor of many months, even years, to show that the symptoms in a case of neurotic break-down have their meaning, serve a purpose, and result from the fortunes of the patient. On the other hand, the efforts of a few hours suffice in proving the same content in a dream product which at first seems incomprehensibly confused, and thereby to confirm all the hypotheses of psychoanalysis, the unconsciousness of psychic processes, the special mechanism which they follow, and the motive forces which manifest themselves in them. And if we associate the thorough analogy in the construction of the dream and the neurotic symptom with the rapidity of transformation which makes of the dreamer an alert and reasonable individual, we gain the certainty that the neurosis also is based only on a change in the balance of the forces of psychic life.

III

GENERAL THEORY OF THE NEUROSES

SIXTEENTH LECTURE

GENERAL THEORY OF THE NEUROSES

Psychoanalysis and Psychiatry

IAM very glad to welcome you back to continue our discussions. I last lectured to you on the psychoanalytic treatment of errors and of the dream. To-day I should like to introduce you to an understanding of neurotic phenomena, which, as you soon will discover, have much in common with both of those topics. But I shall tell you in advance that I cannot leave you to take the same attitude toward me that you had before. At that time I was anxious to take no step without complete reference to your judgment. I discussed much with you, I listened to your objections, in short, I deferred to you and to your "normal common sense." That is no longer possible, and for a very simple reason. As phenomena, the dream and errors were not strange to you. One might say that you had as much experience as I, or that you could easily acquire as much. But neuroses are foreign to you; since you are not doctors yourselves you have had access to them only through what I have told you. Of what use is the best judgment if it is not supported by familiarity with the material in question?

Do not, however, understand this as an announcement of dogmatic lectures which demand your unconditional belief. That would be a gross misunderstanding. I do not wish to convince you. I am out to stimulate your interest and shake your prejudices. If, in consequence of not knowing the facts, you are not in a position to judge, neither should you believe nor condemn. Listen and allow yourselves to be influenced by what I tell you. One cannot be so easily convinced; at least if he comes by convictions without effort, they soon prove to be valueless and unable to hold their own. He only has a right to conviction who has handled the same material for many years and who in so doing has gone through the same new and surprising experiences again and again. Why, in matters of intellect these lightning conversions, these momentary repulsions? Do you not feel that a *coup de foudre*, that love at first sight, originates in quite a different field, namely, in that of the emotions? We do not even demand that our patients should become convinced of and predisposed to psychoanalysis. When they do, they seem suspicious to us. The attitude we prefer in them is one of benevolent scepticism. Will you not also try to let the psychoanalytic conception develop in your mind beside the popular or "psychiatric"? They will influence each other, mutually measure their strength, and some day work themselves into a decision on your part.

On the other hand, you must not think for a moment that what I present to you as the psychoanalytic conception is a purely speculative system. Indeed, it is a sum total of experiences and observations, either their direct expression or their elaboration. Whether this elaboration is done adequately and whether the method is justifiable will be tested in the further progress of the science. After two and a half decades, now that I am fairly advanced in years, I may say that it was particularly difficult, intensive and all-absorbing work which yielded these observations. I have often had the impression that our opponents were unwilling to take into consideration this objective origin of our statements, as if they thought it were only a question of subjective ideas arising haphazard, ideas to which another may oppose his every passing whim. This antagonistic behavior is not entirely comprehensible to me. Perhaps the physician's habit of steering clear of his neurotic patients and listening so very casually to what they have to say allows him to lose sight of the possibility of deriving anything valuable from his patients' communications, and therefore, of making penetrating observations on them. I take this opportunity of promising you that I shall carry on little controversy in the course of my lectures, least of all with individual controversialists. I have never been able to convince myself of the truth of the saying that controversy is the father of all things. I believe that it comes down to us from the Greek sophist philosophy and errs as does the latter through the overvaluation of dialectics. To me, on the contrary, it seems as if the so-called scientific criticism were on the whole unfruitful, quite apart from the fact that it is almost always carried on in a most personal spirit. For my part, up to a few years ago, I could even boast that I had entered into a regular scientific dispute with only one scholar (Lowenfeld, of Munich). The end of this was that we became friends and have remained friends to this day. But I did not repeat this attempt for a long time, because I was not certain that the outcome would be the same.

Now you will surely judge that so to reject the discussion of literature must evidence stubborness, a very special obtuseness against objections, or, as the kindly colloquialisms of science have it, "a complete personal bias." In answer, I would say that should you attain to a conviction by such hard labor, you would thereby derive a certain right to sustain it with some tenacity. Furthermore, I should like to emphasize the fact that I have modified my views on certain important points in the course of my researches, changed them and replaced them by new ones, and that I naturally made a public statement of that fact each time. What has been the result of this frankness? Some paid no attention at all to my self-corrections and even to-day criticize me for assertions which have long since ceased to have the same meaning for me. Others reproach me for just this deviation, and on account of it declare me unreliable. For is anyone who has changed his opinions several times still trustworthy; is not his latest assertion, as well, open to error? At the same time he who holds unswervingly to what he has once said, or cannot be made to give it up quickly enough, is called stubborn and biased. In the face of these contradictory criticisms, what else can one do but be himself and act according to his own dictates? That is what I have decided to do, and I will not allow myself to be restrained from modifying and adapting my theories as the progress of my experience demands. In the basic ideas I have hitherto found nothing to change, and I hope that such will continue to be the case.

Now I shall present to you the psychoanalytic conception of neurotic manifestations. The natural thing for me to do is to connect them to the phenomena we have previously treated, for the sake of their analogy as well as their contrast. I will select as symptomatic an act of frequent occurrence in my office hour. Of course, the analyst cannot do much for those who seek him in his medical capacity, and lay the woes of a lifetime before him in fifteen minutes. His deeper knowledge makes it difficult for him to deliver a snap decision as do other physicians—"There is nothing wrong with you"—and to give the advice, "Go to a watering-place for a while." One of our colleagues, in answer to the question as to what he did with his office patients, said, shrugging his shoulders, that he simply "fines them so many kronen for their mischief-making." So it will not surprise you to hear that even in the case of very busy analysts, the hours for consultation are not very crowded. I have had the ordinary door between my waiting room and my office doubled and strengthened by a covering of felt. The purpose of this little arrangement cannot be doubted. Now it happens over and over again that people who are admitted from my waiting room omit to close the door behind them; in fact, they almost always leave both doors open. As soon as I have noticed this I insist rather gruffly that he or she go back in order to rectify the omission, even though it be an elegant gentleman or a lady in all her finery. This gives an impression of misapplied pedantry. I have, in fact, occasionally discredited myself by such a demand, since the individual concerned was one of those who cannot touch even a door knob, and prefer as well to have their attendants spared this contact. But most frequently I was right, for he who conducts himself in this way, and leaves the door from the waiting room into the physician's consultation room open, belongs to the rabble and deserves to be received inhospitably. Do not, I beg you, defend him until you have heard what follows. For the fact is that this negligence of the patient's only occurs when he has been alone in the waiting room and so leaves an empty room behind him, never when others, strangers, have been waiting with him. If that latter is the case, he knows very well that it is in his interest not to be listened to while he is talking to the physician, and never omits to close both the doors with care.

This omission of the patient's is so predetermined that it becomes neither accidental nor meaningless, indeed, not even unimportant, for, as we shall see, it throws light upon the relation of this patient to the physician. He is one of the great number of those who seek authority, who want to be dazzled, intimidated. Perhaps he had inquired by telephone as to what time he had best call, he had prepared himself to come on a crowd of suppliants somewhat like those in front of a branch milk station. He now enters an empty waiting room which is, moreover, most modestly furnished, and he is disappointed. He must demand reparation from the physician for the wasted respect that he had tendered him, and so he omits to close the door between the reception room and the office. By this, he means to say to the physician: "Oh, well, there is no one here anyway, and probably no one will come as long as I am here." He would also be quite unmannerly and supercilious during the consultation if his presumption were not at once restrained by a sharp reminder.

You will find nothing in the analysis of this little symptomatic act which was not previously known to you. That is to say, it asserts that this act is not accidental, but has a motive, a meaning, a purpose, that it has its assignable connections psychologically, and that it serves as a small indication of a more important psychological process. But above all it implies that the process thus intimated is not known to the consciousness of the individual in whom it takes place, for none of the patients who left the two doors open would have admitted that they meant by this omission to show me their contempt. Some could probably recall a slight sense of disappointment at entering an empty waiting room, but the connection between this impression and the symptomatic act which followed—of these, his consciousness was surely not aware.

Now let us place, side by side with this small analysis of a symptomatic act, an observation on a pathological case. I choose one which is fresh in my mind and which can also be described with relative brevity. A certain measure of minuteness of detail is unavoidable in any such account.

A young officer, home on a short leave of absence, asked me to see his mother-in-law who, in spite of the happiest circumstances, was embittering her own and her people's existence by a senseless idea. I am introduced to a well preserved lady of fifty-three with pleasant, simple manners, who gives the following account without any hesitation: She is most happily married and lives in the country with her husband, who operates a large factory. She cannot say enough for the kind thoughtfulness of her husband. They had married for love thirty years ago, and since then there had never been a shadow, a quarrel or cause for jealousy. Now, even though her two children are well married, the husband and father does not yet want to retire, from a feeling of duty. A year ago there happened the incredible thing, incomprehensible to herself as well. She gave complete credence to an anonymous letter which accused her excellent husband of having an affair with a young girl—and since then her happiness is destroyed. The more detailed circumstances were somewhat as follows: She had a chambermaid with whom she had perhaps too often discussed intimate matters. This girl pursued another young woman with positively malicious enmity because the latter had progressed so much further in life, despite the fact that she was of no better origin. Instead of going into domestic service, the girl had obtained a business training, had entered the factory and in consequence of the short-handedness due to the drafting of the clerks into the army had advanced to a good position. She now lives in the factory itself, meets all the gentlemen socially, and is even addressed as "Miss." The girl who had remained behind in life was of course ready to speak all possible evil of her one-time schoolmate. One day our patient and her chambermaid were talking of an old gentleman who had been visiting at the house, and of whom it was known that he did not live with his wife, but kept another woman as his mistress. She does not know how it happened that she suddenly remarked, "That would be the most awful thing that could happen to me, if I should ever hear that my good husband also had a mistress." The next day she received an anonymous letter through the mail which, in a disguised handwriting, carried this very communication which she had conjured up. She concluded—it seems justifiably—that the letter was the handiwork of her malignant chambermaid, for the letter named as the husband's mistress the self-same woman whom the maid persecuted with her hatred. Our patient, in spite of the fact that she immediately saw through the intrigue and had seen enough in her town to know how little credence such cowardly denunciations deserve, was nevertheless at once prostrated by the letter. She became dreadfully excited and promptly sent for her husband in order to heap the bitterest reproaches upon him. Her husband laughingly denied the accusation and did the best that could be done. He called in the family physician, who was as well the doctor in attendance at the factory, and the latter added his efforts to quiet the unhappy woman. Their further procedure was also entirely reasonable. The chambermaid was dismissed, but the pretended rival was not. Since then, the patient claims she has repeatedly so far calmed herself as no longer to believe the contents of the anonymous letter, but this relief was neither thoroughgoing nor lasting. It was enough to hear the name of the young lady spoken or to meet her on the street in order to precipitate a new attack of suspicion, pain and reproach.

This, now, is the case history of this good woman. It does not need much psychiatric experience to understand that her portrayal of her own case was, if anything, rather too mild in contrast to other nervous patients. The picture, we say, was dissimulated; in reality she had never overcome her belief in the accusation of the anonymous letter.

Now what position does a psychiatrist take toward such a case? We already know what he would do in the case of the symptomatic act of the patient who does not close the doors to the waiting room. He declares it an accident without psychological interest, with which he need not concern himself. But this attitude cannot be maintained toward the pathological case of the jealous woman. The symptomatic act seems no great matter, but the symptom itself claims attention by reason of its gravity. It is bound up with intense subjective suffering while objectively it threatens to break up a home; therefore its claim to psychiatric interest cannot be put aside. The first endeavor of the psychiatrist is to characterize the symptom by some distinctive feature. The idea with which this woman torments herself cannot in itself be called nonsensical, for it does happen that elderly married men have affairs with young girls. But there is something else about it that is nonsensical and incredible. The patient has no reason beyond the declaration in the anonymous letter to believe that her tender and faithful husband belongs to this sort of married men, otherwise not uncommon. She knows that this letter in itself carries no proof; she can satisfactorily explain its origin; therefore she ought to be able to persuade herself that she has no reason to be jealous. Indeed she does this, but in spite of it she suffers every bit as much as she would if she acknowledged this jealousy as fully justified. We are agreed to call ideas of this sort, which are inaccessible to arguments based on logic or on facts, "*obsessions*." Thus the good lady suffers from an "*obsession of jealousy*" that is surely a distinctive characterization for this pathological case.

Having reached this first certainty, our psychiatric interest will have become aroused. If we cannot do away with a delusion by taking reality into account, it can hardly have arisen from reality. But the delusion, what is its origin? There are delusions of the most widely varied content. Why is it that in our case the content should be jealousy? In what types of persons are obsessions liable to occur, and, in particular, obsessions of jealousy? We would like to turn to the psychiatrist with such questions, but here he leaves us in the lurch. There is only one of our queries which he heeds. He will examine the family history of this woman and *perhaps* will give us the answer: "The people who develop obsessions are those in whose families similar and other psychic disturbances have repeatedly occurred." In other words, if this lady develops an obsession she does so because she was predisposed to it by reason of her heredity. That is certainly something, but is it all that we want to know? Is it all that was effective in causing this breakdown? Shall we be content to assume that it is immaterial, accidental and inexplicable why the obsession of jealousy develops rather than any other? And may we also accept this sentence about the dominance of the influence of heredity in its negative meaning, that is, that no matter what experiences came to this human being she was predestined to develop some kind of obsession? You will want to know why scientific psychiatry will give no further explanation. And I reply, "He is a rascal who gives more than he owns." The psychiatrist does not know of any path that leads him further in the explanation of such a case. He must content himself with the diagnosis and a prognosis which, despite a wealth of experience, is uncertain.

Yet, can psychoanalysis do more at this point? Indeed yes! I hope to show you that even in so inaccessible a case as this it can discover something which makes the further understanding possible. May I ask you first to note the apparently insignificant fact that the patient actually provoked the anonymous letter which now supports her delusion. The day before, she announces to the intriguing chambermaid that if her husband were to have an affair with a young girl it would be the worst misfortune that could befall her. By so doing she really gave the maid the idea of sending her the anonymous letter. The obsession thus attains a certain independence from the letter; it existed in the patient beforehand—perhaps as a dread; or was it a wish? Consider, moreover, these additional details yielded by an analysis of only two hours. The patient was indeed most helpful when, after telling her story, she was urged to communicate her further thoughts, ideas and recollections. She declared that nothing came to her mind, that she had already told everything. After two hours the undertaking had really to be given up because she announced that she already felt cured and was sure that the morbid idea would not return. Of course, she said this because of this resistance and her fear of continuing the analysis. In these two hours, however, she had let fall certain remarks which made possible definite interpretation, indeed made it incontestable; and this interpretation throws a clear light on the origin of her obsession of jealousy. Namely, she herself was very much infatuated with a certain young man, the very same son-in-law upon whose urging she had come to consult me professionally.

She knew nothing of this infatuation, or at least only a very little. Because of the existing relationship, it was very easy for this infatuation to masquerade under the guise of harmless tenderness. With all our further experience it is not difficult to feel our way toward an understanding of the psychic life of this honest woman and good mother. Such an infatuation, a monstrous, impossible thing, could not be allowed to become conscious. But it continued to exist and unconsciously exerted a heavy pressure. Something had to happen, some sort of relief had to be found and the mechanism of displacement which so constantly takes part in the origin of obsessional jealousy offered the most immediate mitigation. If not only she, old woman that she was, was in love with a young man but if also her old husband had an affair with a young girl, then she would be freed from the voice of her conscience which accused her of infidelity. The phantasy of her husband's infidelity was thus like a cooling salve on her burning wound. Of her own love she never became conscious, but the reflection of it, which would bring her such advantages, now became compulsive, obsessional and conscious. Naturally all arguments directed against the obsession were of no avail since they were directed only to the reflection, and not to the original force to which it owed its strength and which, unimpeachable, lay buried in the unconscious.

Let us now piece together these fragments to see what a short and impeded psychoanalysis can nevertheless contribute to the understanding of this case. It is assumed of course that our inquiries were carefully conducted, a point which I cannot at this place submit to your judgment. In the first place, the obsession becomes no longer nonsensical nor incomprehensible, it is full of meaning, well motivated and an integral part of the patient's emotional experience. Secondly, it is a necessary reaction toward an unconscious psychological process, revealed in other ways, and it is to this very circumstance that it owes its obsessional nature, that is, its resistance to arguments based on logic or fact. In itself the obsession is something wished for, a kind of consolation. Finally, the experiences underlying the condition are such as unmistakably determine an obsession of jealousy and no other. You will also recognize the part played by the two important analogies in the analysis of the symptomatic act with reference to its meaning and intent and also to its relation to an unconscious factor in the situation.

Naturally, we have not yet answered all the questions which may be put on the basis of this case. Rather the case bristles with further problems of a kind which we have not yet been able to solve in any way, and of others which could not be solved because of the disadvantage of the circumstances under which we were working. For example: why is this happily married woman open to an infatuation for her son-in-law, and why does the relief which could have been obtained in other ways come to her by way of this mirror-image, this projection of her own condition upon her husband? I trust you will not think that it is idle and wanton to open such problems. Already we have much material at our disposal for their possible solution. This woman is in that critical age when her sexual needs undergo a sudden and unwelcome exaggeration. This might in itself be sufficient. In addition, her good and faithful mate may for many years have been lacking in that sufficient sexual capacity which the well-preserved woman needs for her satisfaction. We have learned by experience to know that those very men whose faithfulness is thus placed beyond a doubt are most gentle in their treatment of their wives and unusually forbearing toward their nervous complaints. Furthermore, the fact that it was just the young husband of a daughter who became the object of her abnormal infatuation is by no means insignificant. A strong erotic attachment to the daughter, which in the last analysis leads back to the mother's sexual constitution, will often find a way to live on under such a disguise. May I perhaps remind you in this connection that the relationship between mother and son-in-law has seemed particularly delicate since all time and is one which among primitive peoples gave rise to very powerful taboos and avoidances.[37] It often transgresses our cultural standards positively as well as negatively. I cannot tell you of course which of these three factors were at work in our case; whether two of them only, or whether all of them coöperated, for as you know I did not have the opportunity to continue the analysis beyond two hours.

I realize at this point, ladies and gentlemen, that I have been speaking entirely of things for which your understanding was not prepared. I did this in order to carry through the comparison of psychiatry and psychoanalysis. May I now ask one thing of you? Have you noticed any contradiction between them? Psychiatry does not apply the technical methods of psychoanalysis, and neglects to look for any significance in the content of the obsession. Instead of first seeking out more specific and immediate causes, psychiatry refers us to the very general and remote source—heredity. But does this imply a contradiction, a conflict between them? Do they not rather supplement one another? For does the hereditary factor deny the significance of the experience, is it not rather true that both operate together in the most effective way? You must admit that there is nothing in the nature of psychiatric work which must repudiate psychoanalytic research. Therefore, it is the psychiatrists who oppose psychoanalysis, not psychiatry itself. Psychoanalysis stands in about the same relation to psychiatry as does histology to anatomy. The one studies the outer forms of organs, the other the closer structure of tissues and cells. A contradiction between two types of study, where one simplifies the other, is not easily conceivable. You know that anatomy to-day forms the basis of scientific medicine, but there was a time when the dissection of human corpses to learn the inner structure of the body was as much frowned upon as the practice of psychoanalysis, which seeks to ascertain the inner workings of the human soul, seems proscribed to-day. And presumably a not too distant time will bring us to the realization that a psychiatry which aspires to scientific depth is not possible without a real knowledge of the deeper unconscious processes in the psychic life.

Perhaps this much-attacked psychoanalysis has now found some friends among you who are anxious to see it justify itself as well from another aspect, namely, the therapeutic side. You know that the therapy of psychiatry has hitherto not been able to influence obsessions. Can psychoanalysis perhaps do so, thanks to its insight into the mechanism of these symptoms? No, ladies and gentlemen, it cannot; for the present at least it is just as powerless in the face of these maladies as every other therapy. We can understand what it was that happened within the patient, but we have no means of making the patient himself understand this. In fact, I told you that I could not extend the analysis of the obsession beyond the first steps. Would you therefore assert that analysis is objectionable in such cases because it remains without result? I think not. We have the right, indeed we have the duty to pursue scientific research without regard to an immediate practical effect. Some day, though we do not know when or where, every little scrap of knowledge will have been translated into skill, even into therapeutic skill. If psychoanalysis were as unsuccessful in all other forms of nervous and psychological disease as it is in the case of the obsession, it would nevertheless remain fully justified as an irreplaceable method of scientific research. It is true that we would then not be in a position to practice it, for the human subjects from which we must learn, live and will in their own right; they must have motives of their own in order to assist in the work, but they would deny themselves to us. Therefore let me conclude this session by telling you that there are comprehensive groups of nervous diseases concerning which our better understanding has actually been translated into therapeutic power; moreover, that in disturbances which are most difficult to reach we can under certain conditions secure results which are second to none in the field of internal therapeutics.

SEVENTEENTH LECTURE

GENERAL THEORY OF THE NEUROSES

The Meaning of the Symptoms

IN the last lecture I explained to you that clinical psychiatry concerns itself very little with the form under which the symptoms appear or with the burden they carry, but that it is precisely here that psychoanalysis steps in and shows that the symptom carries a meaning and is connected with the experience of the patient. The meaning of neurotic symptoms was first discovered by J. Breuer in the study and felicitous cure of a case of hysteria which has since become famous (1880-82). It is true that P. Janet independently reached the same result; literary priority must in fact be accorded to the French scholar, since Breuer published his observations more than a decade later (1893-95) during his period of collaboration with me. On the whole it may be of small importance to us who is responsible for this discovery, for you know that every discovery is made more than once, that none is made all at once, and that success is not meted out according to deserts. America is not named after Columbus. Before Breuer and Janet, the great psychiatrist Leuret expressed the opinion that even for the deliria of the insane, if we only understood how to interpret them, a meaning could be found. I confess that for a considerable period of time I was willing to estimate very highly the credit due to P. Janet in the explanation of neurotic symptoms, because he saw in them the expression of subconscious ideas (*idées inconscientes*) with which the patients were obsessed. But since then Janet has expressed himself most conservatively, as though he wanted to confess that the term "subconscious" had been for him nothing more than a mode of speech, a shift, "*une façon de parler,*" by the use of which he had nothing definite in mind. I now no longer understand Janet's discussions, but I believe that he has needlessly deprived himself of high credit.

The neurotic symptoms then have their meaning just like errors and the dream, and like these they are related to the lives of the persons in whom they appear. The importance of this insight into the nature of the symptom can best be brought home to you by way of examples. That it is borne out always and in all cases, I can only assert, not prove. He who gathers his own experience will be convinced of it. For certain reasons, however, I shall draw my instances not from hysteria, but from another fundamentally related and very curious neurosis concerning which I wish to say a few introductory words to you. This so-called compulsion neurosis is not so popular as the widely known hysteria; it is, if I may use the expression, not so noisily ostentatious, behaves more as a private concern of the patient, renounces bodily manifestations almost entirely and creates all its symptoms psychologically. Compulsion neurosis and hysteria are those forms of neurotic disease by the study of which psychoanalysis has been built up, and in whose treatment as well the therapy celebrates its triumphs. Of these the compulsion neurosis, which does not take that mysterious leap from the psychic to the physical, has through psychoanalytic research become more intimately comprehensible and transparent to us than hysteria, and we have come to understand that it reveals far more vividly certain extreme characteristics of the neuroses.

The chief manifestations of compulsion neurosis are these: the patient is occupied by thoughts that in reality do not interest him, is moved by impulses that appear alien to him, and is impelled to actions which, to be sure, afford him no pleasure, but the performance of which he cannot possibly resist. The thoughts may be absurd in themselves or thoroughly indifferent to the individual, often they are absolutely childish and in all cases they are the result of strained thinking, which exhausts the patient, who surrenders himself to them most unwillingly. Against his will he is forced to brood and speculate as though it were a matter of life or death to him. The impulses, which the patient feels within himself, may also give a childish or ridiculous impression, but for the most part they bear the terrifying aspect of temptations to fearful crimes, so that the patient not only denies them, but flees from them in horror and protects himself from actual execution of his desires through inhibitory renunciations and restrictions upon his personal liberty. As a matter of fact he never, not a single time, carries any of these impulses into effect; the result is always that his evasion and precaution triumph. The patient really carries out only very harmless trivial acts, so-called compulsive acts, for the most part repetitions and ceremonious additions to the occupations of every-day life, through which its necessary performances—going to bed, washing, dressing, walking—become long-winded problems of almost insuperable difficulty. The abnormal ideas, impulses and actions are in nowise equally potent in individual forms and cases of compulsion neurosis; it is the rule, rather, that one or the other of these manifestations is the dominating factor and gives the name to the disease; that all these forms, however, have a great deal in common is quite undeniable.

Surely this means violent suffering. I believe that the wildest psychiatric phantasy could not have succeeded in deriving anything comparable, and if one did not actually see it every day, one could hardly bring oneself to believe it. Do not think, however, that you give the patient any help when you coax him to divert himself, to put aside these stupid ideas and to set himself to something useful in the place of his whimsical occupations. This is just what he would like of his own accord, for he possesses all his senses, shares your opinion of his compulsion symptoms, in fact volunteers it quite readily. But he cannot do otherwise; whatever activities actually are released under compulsion neurosis are carried along by a driving energy, such as is probably never met with in normal psychic life. He has only one remedy—to transfer and change. In place of one stupid idea he can think of a somewhat milder absurdity, he can proceed from one precaution and prohibition to another, or carry through another ceremonial. He may shift, but he cannot annul the compulsion. One of the chief characteristics of the sickness is the instability of the symptoms; they can be shifted very far from their original form. It is moreover striking that the contrasts present in all psychological experience are so very sharply drawn in this condition. In addition to the compulsion of positive and negative content, an intellectual doubt makes itself felt that gradually attacks the most ordinary and assured certainties. All these things merge into steadily increasing uncertainty, lack of energy, curtailment of personal liberty, despite the fact that the patient suffering from compulsion neurosis is originally a most energetic character, often of extraordinary obstinacy, as a rule intellectually gifted above the average. For the most part he has attained a desirable stage of ethical development, is overconscientious and more than usually correct. You can imagine that it takes no inconsiderable piece of work to find one's way through this maze of contradictory characteristics and symptoms. Indeed, for the present our only object is to understand and to interpret some symptoms of this disease.

Perhaps in reference to our previous discussions, you would like to know the position of present-day psychiatry to the problems of the compulsion neurosis. This is covered in a very slim chapter. Psychiatry gives names to the various forms of compulsion, but says nothing further concerning them. Instead it emphasizes the fact that those who show these symptoms are degenerates. That yields slight satisfaction, it is an ethical judgment, a condemnation rather than an explanation. We are led to suppose that it is in the unsound that all these peculiarities may be found. Now we do believe that persons who develop such symptoms must differ fundamentally from other people. But we would like to ask, are they more "degenerate" than other nervous patients, those suffering, for instance, from hysteria or other diseases of the mind? The characterization is obviously too general. One may even doubt whether it is at all justified, when one learns that such symptoms occur in excellent men and women of especially great and universally recognized ability. In general we glean very little intimate knowledge of the great men who serve us as models. This is due both to their own discretion and to the lying propensities of their biographers. Sometimes, however, a man is a fanatic disciple of truth, such as Emile Zola, and then we hear from him the strange compulsion habits from which he suffered all his life.[38]

Psychiatry has resorted to the expedient of speaking of "superior degenerates." Very well—but through psychoanalysis we have learned that these peculiar compulsion symptoms may be permanently removed just like any other disease of normal persons. I myself have frequently succeeded in doing this.

I will give you two examples only of the analysis of compulsion symptoms, one, an old observation, which cannot be replaced by anything more complete, and one a recent study. I am limiting myself to such a small number because in an account of this nature it is necessary to be very explicit and to enter into every detail.

A lady about thirty years old suffered from the most severe compulsions. I might indeed have helped her if caprice of fortune had not destroyed my work—perhaps I will yet have occasion to tell you about it. In the course of each day the patient often executed, among others, the following strange compulsive act. She ran from her room into an adjoining one, placed herself in a definite spot beside a table which stood in the middle of the room, rang for her maid, gave her a trivial errand to do, or dismissed her without more ado, and then ran back again. This was certainly not a severe symptom of disease, but it still deserved to arouse curiosity. Its explanation was found, absolutely without any assistance on the part of the physician, in the very simplest way, a way to which no one can take exception. I hardly know how I alone could have guessed the meaning of this compulsive act, or have found any suggestion toward its interpretation. As often as I had asked the patient: "Why do you do this? Of what use is it?" she had answered, "I don't know." But one day after I had succeeded in surmounting a grave ethical doubt of hers she suddenly saw the light and related the history of the compulsive act. More than ten years prior she had married a man far older than herself, who had proved impotent on the bridal night. Countless times during the night he had run from his room to hers to repeat the attempt, but each time without success. In the morning he said angrily: "It is enough to make one ashamed before the maid who does the beds," and took a bottle of red ink that happened to be in the room, and poured its contents on the sheet, but not on the place where such a stain would have been justifiable. At first I did not understand the connection between this reminiscence and the compulsive act in question, for the only agreement I could find between them was in the running from one room into another,—possibly also in the appearance of the maid. Then the patient led me to the table in the second room and let me discover a large spot on the cover. She explained also that she placed herself at the table in such a way that the maid could not miss seeing the stain.

Now it was no longer possible to doubt the intimate relation of the scene after her bridal night and her present compulsive act, but there were still a number of things to be learned about it.

In the first place, it is obvious that the patient identifies herself with her husband, she is acting his part in her imitation of his running from one room into the other. We must then admit—if she holds to this role—that she replaces the bed and sheet by table and cover. This may seem arbitrary, but we have not studied dream symbolism in vain. In dreams also a table which must be interpreted as a bed, is frequently seen. "Bed and board" together represent married life, one may therefore easily be used to represent the other.

The evidence that the compulsive act carries meaning would thus be plain; it appears as a representation, a repetition of the original significant scene. However, we are not forced to stop at this semblance of a solution; when we examine more closely the relation between these two people, we shall probably be enlightened concerning something of wider importance, namely, the purpose of the compulsive act. The nucleus of this purpose is evidently the summoning of the maid; to her she wishes to show the stain and refute her husband's remark: "It is enough to shame one before the maid." He—whose part she is playing—therefore feels no shame before the maid, hence the stain must be in the right place. So we see that she has not merely repeated the scene, rather she has amplified it, corrected it and "turned it to the good." Thereby, however, she also corrects something else,—the thing which was so embarrassing that night and necessitated the use of the red ink— impotence. The compulsive act then says: "No, it is not true, he did not have to be ashamed before the maid, he was not impotent." After the manner of a dream she represents the fulfillment of this wish in an overt action, she is ruled by the desire to help her husband over that unfortunate incident.

Everything else that I could tell you about this case supports this clue more specifically; all that we otherwise know about her tends to strengthen this interpretation of a compulsive act incomprehensible in itself. For years the woman has lived separated from her husband and is struggling with the intention to obtain a legal divorce. But she is by no means free from him; she forces herself to remain faithful to him, she retires from the world to avoid temptation; in her imagination she excuses and idealizes him. The deepest secret of her malady is that by means of it she shields her husband from malicious gossip, justifies her separation from him, and renders possible for him a comfortable separate life. Thus the analysis of a harmless compulsive act leads to the very heart of this case and at the same time reveals no inconsiderable portion of the secret of the compulsion neurosis in general. I shall be glad to have you dwell upon this instance, as it combines conditions that one can scarcely demand in other cases. The interpretation of the symptoms was discovered by the patient herself in one flash, without the suggestion or interference of the analyst. It came about by the reference to an experience, which did not, as is usually the case, belong to the half-forgotten period of childhood, but to the mature life of the patient, in whose memory it had remained unobliterated. All the objections which critics ordinarily offer to our interpretation of symptoms fail in this case. Of course, we are not always so fortunate.

And one thing more! Have you not observed how this insignificant compulsive act initiated us into the intimate life of the invalid? A woman can scarcely relate anything more intimate than the story of her bridal night, and is it without further significance that we just happened to come on the intimacies of her sexual life? It might of course be the result of the selection I have made in this instance. Let us not judge too quickly and turn our attention to the second instance, one of an entirely different kind, a sample of a frequently occurring variety, namely, the sleep ritual.

A nineteen-year old, well-developed, gifted girl, an only child, who was superior to her parents in education and intellectual activity, had been wild and mischievous in her childhood, but has become very nervous during the last years without any apparent outward cause. She is especially irritable with her mother, always discontented, depressed, has a tendency toward indecision and doubt, and is finally forced to confess that she can no longer walk alone on public squares or wide thoroughfares. We shall not consider at length her complicated condition, which requires at least two diagnoses—agoraphobia and compulsion neurosis. We will dwell only upon the fact that this girl has also developed a sleep ritual, under which she allows her parents to suffer much discomfort. In a certain sense, we may say that every normal person has a sleep ritual, in other words that he insists on certain conditions, the absence of which hinders him from falling asleep; he has created certain observances by which he bridges the transition from waking to sleeping and these he repeats every evening in the same manner. But everything that the healthy person demands in order to obtain sleep is easily understandable and, above all, when external conditions necessitate a change, he adapts himself easily and without loss of time. But the pathological ritual is rigid, it persists by virtue of the greatest sacrifices, it also masks itself with a reasonable justification and seems, in the light of superficial observation, to differ from the normal only by exaggerated pedantry. But under closer observation we notice that the mask is transparent, for the ritual covers intentions that go far beyond this reasonable justification, and other intentions as well that are in direct contradiction to this reasonable justification. Our patient cites as the motive of her nightly precautions that she must have quiet in order to sleep; therefore she excludes all sources of noise. To accomplish this, she does two things

62659224R00097

Made in the USA
Middletown, DE
24 August 2019